TRAINING
THE OVER 50s

FITNESS PROFESSIONALS

TRAINING THE OVER 50s

SUE GRIFFIN

developing specific programmes for older clients

A & C BLACK • LONDON

Thanks to Fitness Professionals Ltd (www.fitpro.com) for supporting the Fitness Professionals series.

First published in 2006 by A & C Black Publishers Ltd
38 Soho Square, London W1D 3HB
www.acblack.com

Copyright © 2006 by Sue Griffin

ISBN-10: 0 7136 7201 3
ISBN-13: 978 0 7136 7201 5

A CIP catalogue record for this book is available from the British Library.

Typeset in 10½ on 12pt Baskerville BE Regular by Palimpsest Book Production Limited, Polmont, Stirlingshire.

Cover images © John Henley/CORBIS

A & C Black uses paper produced with elemental chlorine-free pulp, harvested from managed sustainable forests.

Printed and bound in Great Britain by Biddles Ltd, Kings Lynn.

Dedicated to the loving memory of my dear dad, Tom Griffin, who always told me that I could, and also to my mum, Audrey, with love and gratitude, who always knew that I would … and made sure that I did!

ACKNOWLEDGEMENTS

With sincere thanks to the following people whose guidance, support and willingness to share their specialist knowledge made it possible to write this book.

Ruth Barlow, Clinical Specialist Respiratory Therapist at Broomfield Hospital; Carol Wells, Falls Co-ordinator; Liz Skidmore, Cardiac Nurse Specialist; Sheetra Rodrigo, Physiotherapist Stroke Specialist; Sharon Eaglestone, BHSc, MCSP SRP, New Century Physiotherapy Ltd, Laindon; Robert Foss, Commissioning Editor at A&C Black Publishers.

A special thanks to Marion Cooper, Senior GP Referral Consultant at Harlow Sportcentre whose expertise and practical knowledge was generously shared and weaves through every aspect of Part Three.

Thanks also to Harlow Sportcentre and their members who are the spirit and inspiration of this book.

And finally for T … thank you for giving me space and being there.

CONTENTS

INTRODUCTION

Did you know that regular physical activity could delay the normal ageing process by 10–20 years? Being on the wrong side of 40 myself, I was very pleased to learn that. If, however, you're not on the wrong side of 40, and are in denial that ageing does actually happen, then think on … and read on! If you take time to ponder the reality of being able to slow down ageing and what it means, is a very powerful message, you and your skills as an instructor can *really* enhance people's lives. In the first few pages of Part One you will discover the extent of the opportunity you now have to improve the lives of older adults. At present in the UK, there are more people over the age of 60 than there are under the age of 16, and life expectancy has nearly doubled in the last century.

This guide has been written to provide you with the information you need to apply your existing knowledge of health and fitness to the physical, psychological and wellbeing needs of older adults. The contents also align to *Skills Active National Standards Unit D441* requirements for adapting physical activity to the needs of older adults and are set out in Table 0.1 (on page xi). Your skills as an exercise trainer have never been in more demand and older adults need and *want* the knowledge you can give them. To help you expand your understanding of how and why we age, Part One looks at the theories of ageing and the physical changes that occur as we get older. Having some knowledge about what each of the theories has to say will give you a stronger basis on which to develop your understanding of how you can help older adults age 'successfully'. There is no escaping the physical changes that occur but, now we know the good news, we can certainly slow things down. In Chapter 2 the physiological effects of ageing are summarised and you will be able to quickly assess how ageing affects exercise ability.

Throughout the book I encourage you to consider how an exercise programme can enhance the daily living of your clients. In Part Two the principles and components of fitness are applied to both functional and balance training, which will enable you to apply real life needs and purpose to an exercise programme. There are guides that set out the life advantages of specific exercise, and you can use this knowledge to motivate your clients and personalise their programme. There is also information and guidance on what kind of exercise and training is particularly suitable for older adults.

Most adults over the age of 65 will have one or more chronic conditions and Part Three has been set out to enable quick and easy reference to the information you need to know about a client's condition before you recommend an exercise programme. Each condition is broken down into sub catergories covering the following topics:

- what the condition is
- exercise recommendations
- special considerations and screening guidelines
- client care and education
- adaptations and modifications.

There is an exercise recommendation summary at the end of each section that you can photocopy. This will be very useful if you have a client with more than one condition and you want to review the information together.

Working with older adults will draw on all your skills as a trainer and require you to develop professionally and personally. The challenges of developing exercise and training programmes for clients with one or more chronic conditions will need creativity and ingenuity as well as the knowledge you find in this guide. For those on the outside, working with older adults may appear dull, but in reality you get to meet fascinating characters whose life experiences can teach, amuse and enhance your appreciation of who you are and where you want to be.

There is an opportunity to make a real difference, and the enhanced quality of life you bring to others is returned in spades to yourself through work and life satisfaction. Part Four summarises skills that can enhance your work with older adults and also gives you insights into how you can motivate and inspire them along the way. I have seen people's lives transformed as they nurture themselves back to health after a heart attack or an operation. The friendships and care found in a group can help ease the sorrow of bereavement. I've witnessed the frustration and tears of chronic pain and also the pride of accomplishment and the determination to overcome physical limitations. There is also such a willingness to laugh and have fun.

I wish you fulfilment in your training of older adults and I hope this book supports and guides your own personal development and style to enhance the lives of older adults.

Sue Griffin
February 2006

Table 0.1	National training standards for working with older adults	
What do you need to know?	*What you will find*	*Page reference*
Overview of ageing and physical activity	• demographics • definitions and theories of ageing • physical activity and ageing research • physical activity, disease prevention and functional fitness.	2 3 7 8
Physiological aspects of physical activity and ageing. Physiological and biological – mechanical changes and their effects on mobility and exercise response.	• skeletal system changes • muscular system changes • respiratory system changes • cardiovascular system changes • nervous system changes	20 17 18 12 22
Psychological and socio-cultural aspects of physical activity and ageing.	• understanding older adults • attitude and motivation • physical activity and wellbeing	137 144 144
Screening assessment and goal setting.	• legal and ethical responsibilities • collecting and interpreting information • when to refer on to a health care professional and the information they will need • assessments for evaluation of older clients' physical ability and readiness to exercise • responding to barriers to physical activity • goals of older adults	69 147 139 150 145 149 &151
Programme design and management of older adults	• FITT principles of exercise • programme component guidelines • motivation and adherence • reassessment and evaluation	37 34 144 147
Programme design for older adults with low risk non-referred medical conditions. Common medical conditions and the effect of physical activity, i.e. functional limitations and adaptation of exercise.	• arthritis • osteoporosis • lower back pain • diabetes • stroke • COPD • coronary heart disease • hypertension	82 102 92 109 114 118 126 131

Table 0.1	National training standards for working with older adults cont.	
What do you need to know?	What you will find	Page reference
Teaching and instructing skills	• communication, planning and instruction for maximum effectiveness	137
Client safety and first aid	• when to cease exercise • emergency action plan • the environment	139

WHY TRAIN THE OLDER ADULT?

PART **ONE**

UNDERSTANDING THE AGEING PROCESS

Ageing is inevitable, and affects every single one of us. No one can escape this fact.

I begin with a statement of the obvious, as it is something we tend to ignore because it can make us feel uncomfortable. We bury thoughts of ageing like the cigarette smoker ignores their risk of lung cancer and the obese person who keeps piling on the pounds. And like cancer and obesity, the ageing population is a health issue that could have far-reaching effects on our economy, health and medical resources for current and future generations.

This means there is an opportunity for the fitness professional to use their skills and knowledge to make a difference to the quality of life for the older adults in their community, and also know that forearmed is forewarned. Your younger clients can only gain from understanding the ageing process, and with that extra intelligence you can be reassured that you and your clients can learn how to age successfully and well.

Age structure in the UK

In 1901 the average life expectancy was 45 years for men and 49 years for women. In 2002 the average life expectancy had risen to 76 years for men and 81 years for women.

We are living in an ageing world and the figures from the last census tell us there are more people over the age of 60 than there are under the age of 16. Life expectancy for both men and women has continued to rise. As a result, older people make up an increasing proportion of the population and projections suggest that life expectancy of older adults will increase by a further three years by 2020. National statistics show that there were 19.8 million people aged 50 and over in the United Kingdom in 2002. This shows a 24 per cent increase over 40 years, from 16 million in 1961. Future growth is predicted to increase by a further 37 per cent by 2031 when there will be close to 27 million people aged 50 and over. The reason for an ageing population is a combination of fewer births leading to fewer young people, as well as a decline in mortality of both the young and older people.

Many older people live active and healthy lives for many years over the age of 50, but for those who have chronic conditions the pain and fear of harming themselves will be a major barrier to increasing activity levels. This can prevent older adults from participating in activities that could ease their symptoms, prevent further deterioration of their condition and the onset of other health problems that are the outcome of a sedentary lifestyle. The impact of an ageing population on our community is already draining NHS resources, creating stress and strain for families who care for elderly parents and, most of all, reducing the quality of life for older members of society. As fitness professionals we can respond to our ageing society by applying our skills and knowledge of exercise and fitness to the older adult.

Research by Age Concern has shown that adults aged 55 and above are eager to take up regular exercise and adopt a healthier lifestyle in order to stay fitter for longer. Further evidence of older adults' commitment to active living comes from a survey by the YMCA Montreal and the University of Calgary entitled *Towards a New Perspective from Ageing to Ageing Well*, which examined the attitudes of 4,675 members towards regular physical exercise in three age groups; 45–54, 55–64 and 65-plus. The results showed that all three age groups were equally confident in their ability to keep exercising, but the 65-plus age group was far more motivated to maintain their current workout rate than their younger counterparts. It also shows that older adults will stick with a physical activity programme if it improves their quality of life.

The needs of the ageing population creates an opportunity for fitness professionals to broaden their knowledge and develop the skills that will help older adults reduce their risk of, or slow the progression of, chronic diseases and frailty in old age. It will allow older adults to live a more fulfilled life in all areas of well being, including emotionally, intellectually, socially, spiritually and vocationally as well as physically. As Dr Tish Doyle-Baker, Clinical Exercise Physiologist at the University of Calgary, points out: 'a fit mature adult is more independent, is psychologically better equipped to make decisions about their health and has far more opportunities to expand their personal talent and give back to society'.

The science and study of ageing

Gerontology is the scientific study of the problems of ageing in all aspects – clinical, biological, historical and sociological. The increasing demand for knowledge to understand the effects of activity on ageing has led to the development of a new study discipline called Gerokinesiology. This combines combining *gero,* the root of the word *gerontology,* and *kinesiology,* the study of the movement of body parts.

Gerokinesiology is an area of study within the larger discipline of kinesiology that focuses on understanding how physical activity influences all aspects of health and wellbeing in the older adult population and the ageing process in general.

The ageing process – definitions

There are three main definitions of ageing:

- chronological
- biological
- functional.

The following is a summary of the theories of ageing that will give you a broader understanding of the current thinking about why we age, and what is meant by 'successful' ageing. People age differently, and these individual differences need to be taken into account when assessing the health and fitness needs of older adults. The theories of ageing attempt to understand why and how people age. Although individuals can share physical signs of ageing (such as greying hair, wrinkles or skin changes), the onset of diseases and chronic conditions can be influenced by other factors and are therefore less predictable. There is an increased likelihood of a disease or chronic condition for those over 65 years of age, and this likelihood increases further with age. The theories of ageing help us have an understanding of what influences the ageing process. By looking at each of the theories and considering how they can influence an individual with regard to their health and fitness, you are in a much better position to develop a safe and effective exercise programme.

As a starting point, **chronological** age

identifies the person as an older adult and with that comes the recognition that you may be dealing with a vulnerable person or group that needs detailed screening before they start exercising. **Functional** age can provide a measure of ability and fitness level, and provide a basis on which to build an effective exercise programme. The **biological and genetic** theories consider influences such as hereditary and physical changes that occur with age, and influence the way **FITT** principles of exercise (see page 37) are adapted for the older adult. The psychological and social theories provide an understanding of what influences the inner drives of a person; what they think and feel, their beliefs and values and the decisions they make with regard to being active or sedentary.

What is ageing?

The most typical way to define age is by *chronological age* – the number of years or months since birth. However, chronological age is an inadequate measure of age when you compare the functional ability of people in the same age group. For example, if you compare the different growth spurts of children, you will find that they do not grow at the same rate. Some mature and develop faster than others, some naturally have greater physical capabilities, whilst other may be more academic or artistic. There are many variables, such as genetics, social influence, education, nutrition and peers. Two children of the same age do not necessarily have the same abilities or interests. Likewise, we cannot assume that all older adults are the same and will all have the same needs, leisure interests and physical abilities.

Functional age

Functional age compares the fitness of individuals of the same age and gender. For example, a man of 65 could have the aerobic endurance of a 45–60 year old in a fitness test, and therefore his functional age regarding aerobic endurance would be 45–60. If there are functional limitations as a result of illness or inactivity this will affect functional ability to perform everyday tasks (for example walking, stair climbing or getting out of a chair) and can lead to a downward spiral of decline as a result of prolonged physical activity.

Spirduso (1995) divided physical function into the following five levels:

1. physically elite
2. physically fit
3. physically independent
4. physically frail
5. physically dependent.

This Hierarchy of Physical Function (see fig. 1.1 opposite) gives the instructor an extra tool following the initial 'physical activity readiness questionnaire' (Par Q) to broaden their understanding of their client's level and needs.

Biological age

Biological age defines age by the body processes and body systems that prevent the body from repairing and regenerating, which leads to disease and disability. The biological theories below and the physiological changes described in Chapter 5 of this part will provide a fuller explanation.

Theories of ageing

Successful ageing

Successful ageing refers to the likelihood of retaining physical fitness, functional independence and psychological wellbeing into old age. The indicators of successful ageing are longevity and a reduced risk of chronic disease such as cardiovascular disease, diabetes, osteoporosis, sarcopenia (loss of muscle mass),

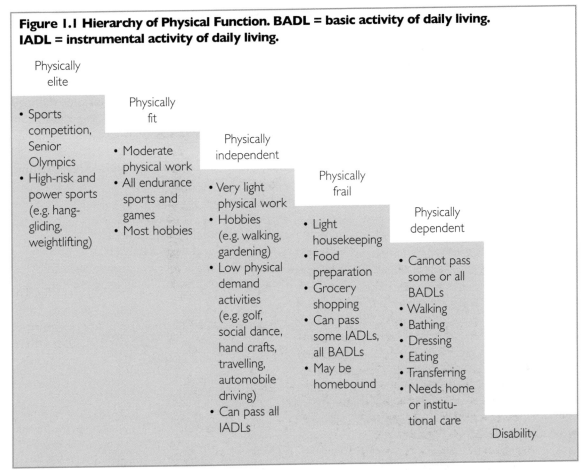

Figure 1.1 Hierarchy of Physical Function. BADL = basic activity of daily living. IADL = instrumental activity of daily living.

From W.W. Spirduso, 1995, *Physical Dimensions of Aging*, page 339, figure 12.5 " 1995 by Waneen W. Spirduso. Reprinted with permission from Human Kinetics (Champaign, IL).

and mobility problems. The following is a summary of the theories of ageing that help to broaden your understanding of the ageing process, so that you can direct your clients towards a path of successful ageing.

Biological theories of ageing

The biological theories of ageing, which include *genetic* and *cellular damage* theories, are more complex and should not be considered fact, as no single theory can fully explain the ageing process. However, biological theorists do provide a broader perspective to try and understand the extent to which an individual's biological age compares to the average person's chronological age. For example, someone who is active and ageing well may have a biological age ten years younger that their chronological age, or a person who has a chronic condition and lives a sedentary lifestyle may be biologically older than they are chronologically.

Genetic theories

There is a lack of agreement as to how much genetics determines the ageing process, but it is generally believed to be in the region of 30–40 per cent (Rowe and Kahn, 1998). Genetic theories focus on how the role of heredity affects the rate at which we age. Although only a few genes actually control the rate of ageing, thousands of genes are responsible for the development of chronic conditions.

Deoxyribonucleic acid (DNA) forms the chemical make up of the human gene and, according to Medveder (1981), ageing of the body occurs as a result of the gradual breakdown of DNA sequences within the cells that leads to incomplete cell reproduction. The *Hayflick Limit Theory* (1961) demonstrates that a cell will only divide a limited number of times (approximately 50), and then it suddenly stops dividing and dies. It has since been discovered that not all cells divide at the same rate. For example, cells of the immune system and endocrine systems divide very few times, while neurons and muscle cells do not divide at all. The implication of this is that people can die of disease before they reach the maximum limit of cell life.

Cellular or damage theories

Cell damage theories of ageing focus on the accumulation of cell damage. The cells are damaged as a result of an accumulation of DNA errors or cross linkages and waste products such as glucose or free radicals within the cells. The most commonly proposed theory of cellular ageing is *Free Radical Theory* (Harman 1956).

A free radical is a highly unstable molecule of oxygen with an uneven number of *electrons* in its outer shell. An unpaired electron is highly unstable and attempts to link up with other molecules, which initiates a destructive chain reaction. In a healthy person, free radical production provides the energy needed for daily living and kills bacterial invaders.

However, excessive free radicals can cause harmful oxidation that is damaging to cell metabolism and correct cell division. Free radicals are especially damaging to the cardiovascular, neuromuscular and endocrine systems. The accumulation of cellular damage increases the risk of diseases such as cardiovascular disease, diabetes and cancer.

Furthermore, a *cross linkage* of fibres is thought to be caused by an increase in free radical oxidation, and molecules of connective tissue (elastin and protein collagen) become intertwined or cross linked, which results in reduced flexibility and range of motion and changes in the skins elasticity. The good news is that leading an active life and eating a healthy diet seems to prevent, or delay, cross-linking.

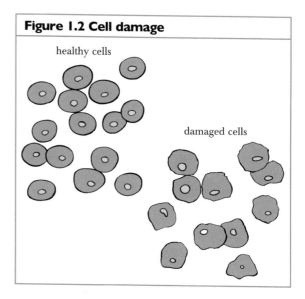

Figure 1.2 Cell damage

healthy cells

damaged cells

Psychological and social theories of ageing

In a similar way that people of the same chronological age can differ biologically, it is also likely that there will be variations in psychological and social age (Schroots & Burren, 1990).

Table 1.1	The following factors determine how we age psychologically
Intelligence	The ability to learn and adapt to new environments, the ability to think non-verbally, knowledge of important facts in your culture.
Cognitive capacity	Mental processing and speed, the ability to solve problems, memory.
Self-efficacy	The belief in your capabilities to handle situations and tasks in life.
Self-esteem	The feelings you hold about yourself.
Personal control	The belief in your ability to exert control in your life.
Coping style	How you adapt to transitions and handle daily hassles and crises.
Resilience	The ability to overcome adversity.

The psychological and social considerations are discussed further and in more detail in Chapter 2.

According to Bandura (1997), a person's self-efficacy is critical for ageing well because it influences thought patterns and emotional reactions, lifestyle choices and behaviours when confronting obstacles throughout life. Through empathic and supportive instruction and guidance, you can work with your older clients towards achievable goals, and increase their self-efficacy and self-esteem so that they experience a new sense of wellbeing and reap the benefits of regular exercise.

The most widely accepted social theory of age is the *activity theory*, which simply states that people who stay engaged in mental and physical activities throughout their life tend to age in a healthier and happier way (Fisher, 1995; Lemon, Bengtson & Peterson, 1972). Social age can also refer to the sometimes rigid expectations of what is appropriate behaviour for a person of a particular age (Rose 1972; Mcgrath & Kelly 1985). Therefore, it is important to be aware of the effects that social roles and expectations have on the lifestyle choices of the older person. For example, many older people consider it undignified to be seen physically exerting themselves in public. The instructor's role is to put the individual at ease, respect their dignity and create a fun, sociable and relaxed atmosphere. Successful ageing depends on environmental and social influences as well as physical and psychological attributes. Ageing is influenced by genetic inheritance, gender and life events, although cultural influences, access to health and social services, personal lifestyle choices and economic status have a large part to play, and are also indicators of how successfully a person will age.

The benefits of physical activity

It is now much more common to see older adults of all age groups working out in the gym, whereas 10 or 15 years ago it would have been a laughable idea to imagine seeing your grandmother lifting weights! The fitness industry has come a long way towards making itself open and accessible to more people, and the knowledge that regular exercise can both alleviate and prevent chronic conditions is much more widespread.

The Government is also taking a leading role in helping to educate and steer people towards making healthier lifestyle choices, including specific recommendations for older adults. The Chief Medical Officer (CMO) has summarised the evidence on the benefits that physical activity has on health. In his report he states that: 'At least 30 minutes of at least moderate intensity physical activity on five or more days a week reduces the risk of premature death from cardiovascular disease and some cancers, significantly reduces the risk of type II diabetes, and can also improve psychological wellbeing.'

Table 1.2 below summarises the key points and key benefits of physical activity for older adults, as outlined in the Chief Medical Officer's Report.

Table 1.2	At least five a week – evidence on the impact of physical activity and its relationship to health
Key Points	Key Benefits
The beneficial effects of physical activity on cardiovascular disease, type II diabetes and obesity are evident for older people (as well as other age groups).	• Physical activity helps to improve several risk factors for cardiovascular disease, including raised blood pressure, adverse blood lipid profiles and insulin resistance. • Exercise-based cardiac rehabilitation programmes for patients with coronary heart disease are generally effective in reducing cardiac deaths and lead to important reductions in all-cause mortality. Treatment with exercise may also be effective in the rehabilitation of people with stroke. • Physically active people have a 33–50 per cent lower risk of developing type II diabetes compared with inactive people. • Among people with type II diabetes, regular moderate-intensity physical activity carried out three times a week can produce small but significant improvements in blood glucose control. Both aerobic and resistance programmes produce similar benefits. • Moderate to high levels of physical fitness appears to reduce the risk of all-cause mortality in patients with type II diabetes.
Regular lifestyle activity is particularly important for older people for the maintenance of mobility and independent living.	• Physical activity can increase bone mineral density in adolescents, maintain it in young adults and slow its decline in old age. • Physical activity in later life can delay the progression of osteoporosis (although it can't reverse advanced bone loss).

Table 1.2	At least five a week – evidence on the impact of physical activity and its relationship to health cont.
Key Points	*Key Benefits*
	• Physical activity can have beneficial effects for people with osteoarthritis, including those who have joint replacement (although too much physical activity can be detrimental).
Strength training exercise can improve muscle strength, which is important for daily living tasks such as walking or getting up from a chair.	• Physical activity can slow down the loss of muscle mass, but cannot halt or reverse it. • Physical strength training using external weight or body weight has been shown to be highly effective in increasing or preserving muscle strength, even into old age. • Strength training programmes involving 2–3 sessions per week with loads greater that 65 per cent of 1 RM (1 rep max) have produced significant improvements in muscle strength in older people.
Physical activity – particularly training to improve strength, balance and co-ordination – has also been found to be highly effective in reducing the incidence of falls.	• Physical activity programmes can help reduce the risk of falling, and therefore fractures, among older people. • In programmes combining strength, balance and endurance training the risk of a fall was reduced by 10 per cent; programmes with balance training alone reduced the risk by 25 per cent and Tai Chi also reduced the risk by 25 per cent.
Physical activity can help improve the emotional and mental wellbeing of older people. It is associated with a reduced risk of developing depressive symptoms, and can be effective in treating depression and enhancing mood.	• Physical activity can help people feel better, as reflected in improved mood and reduced state and trait anxiety. It can help people feel better about themselves through improved physical self perceptions and can improve self-esteem.
Physical activity may improve at least some aspects of cognitive function, which are important to tasks of daily living. It is also associated with reduced risk of developing problems of cognitive impairment in old age.	• Better cognitive performance in older age – particularly in those tasks that are attention demanding and rapid – is associated with increased aerobic fitness, physical activity and sport participation. Those with higher aerobic levels of activity and sports participation are better able to manage those tasks.

AGE RELATED PHYSIOLOGICAL CHANGES

2

Our body begins to age at the moment we are conceived, and physiological change is a continuous and constant process. The physical development from infancy through to adolescence is well understood. However, *why* and *how* we age is less predictable and depends on a number of factors. Although there are changes that typically occur with age, some systems of the body age earlier than others, and they all age uniquely according to the individual. There are organs such as the liver, skin and bone marrow that are able to regenerate and renew lost cells through a process called *hyperplasia* (where the number of cells increases). Other organs such as nerves, muscles, the heart and the lens of the eye will *atrophy* if damaged or unused (where cells and organs shrink in size or form scar tissue).

At its most basic level all living tissue is made up of cells. The cells make up the different organs in the body that form the four basic types of tissue (see figure 2.1 opposite):

1. connective tissue
2. muscle tissue
3. nerve tissue
4. epithelial tissue (the skin and lining of the passages inside the body).

All cells change with age and fatty substances (lipids) and waste (lipofuscin) collect in cells, making it more difficult to absorb the oxygen and nutrients needed to get rid of waste products and carbon dioxide. This causes the connective tissue between the joints to become increasingly stiff, and as a result an organ becomes more rigid and the joints become less flexible. Changes to the organs happen over a long period of time and the detrimental effects

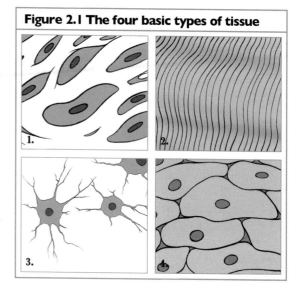

Figure 2.1 The four basic types of tissue

may not be picked up until health problems begin to surface as acute or chronic conditions.

- **acute condition** describes a disease of rapid onset, severe symptoms and brief duration.
- **chronic condition** describes a disease of long duration involving slow changes, and usually a gradual onset. Chronic conditions and chronic pain are described in detail in part three.

Chronic conditions of the cardiovascular, metabolic, musculoskeletal and neurological systems begin to surface with age, and are a major cause of physiological decline (Masoro, 2001). The decline in any system of the body tends to have an affect on other systems, which will increase the risk of disability and frailty in older adults.

The following section summarises the changes in the systems to help you adjust your programme design and expectations about exercise performance.

Changes in metabolism

At any age, the principle of energy in and energy out applies – calories consumed must be used as energy, or they will be stored as fat. For older clients wishing to maintain or lose some weight, they need to have an understanding of their personal metabolism so they can balance the food they consume with their basal metabolic rate (BMR). The BMR is the minimum calories needed to maintain body functions – any calories used for daily activity and exercise should be added to the BMR. From the age of 20 there is a decline in BMR at a rate of 1–2 per cent per decade.

It is also important that your older client is aware of the significance of body composition and how changes in fat and lean tissue will affect BMR, and consequently body weight. Research has shown that older adult body composition decreases in lean body mass, and increases in body fat. According to the research of Evans and Rosenberg (1992), and Forbes (1976), men and women lose more than five pounds of lean body mass (mostly muscle) every decade of life due to disuse. According to another study by Evans Rosenberg (1992) and Keyes *et al.* (1973), a five pound reduction in muscle can result in a 3–5 per cent decrease of BMR per decade. In general, your older client will be completely unaware that a loss of muscle will lower their BMR, or how the calories that were once metabolised by muscles go into fat stores.

However, despite the decline in BMR in older adults there is also plenty of evidence suggesting that a combination of aerobic and strength training can increase lean mass and reduce body fat of older adults aged 40–89 years old. This is good news for the older adult who, with the help of a strength training programme, does not have to resign themselves to weight gain and bigger clothes for the rest of their lives! As the study in the box below shows, exercise can help your older clients to rediscover, or maybe discover for the first time, that they can beat the BMR clock!

A large-scale study conducted at the South Shore YMCA (Westcott and Guy, 1996) compared the results of young, middle, and older adults following an eight-week training programme consisting of 30 minutes of strength exercise and 20 minutes of endurance exercise.

The 1,132 participants in this study included 238 young adults (21 to 40 years), 553 middle-aged adults (41 to 60 years), and 341 older adults (61 to 80 years). All of the three age groups began the programme with similar bodyweights (172.7 to 179.9 lbs) and similar per cent fat readings (25.6 to 27.2 per cent).

After eight weeks of exercise:

- the 21 to 40 year-olds lowered their bodyweight by 2.6 pounds and their body fat by 2.3 per cent. Body composition changes were a loss of 4.9 pounds of fat weight and an increase of 2.3 pounds of lean weight.
- the 41 to 60 year-olds decreased their bodyweight by 2.0 pounds and their body fat by 2.1 per cent. Body composition changes were a loss of 4.4 pounds of fat weight and an increase of 2.3 pounds of lean weight.
- the 61 to 80 year-olds reduced their bodyweight by 1.7 pounds and their body fat by 2 per cent. Body composition changes were a loss of 4.1 pounds of fat weight and an increase of 2.4 pounds of lean weight.

How to work out body composition, BMR, and daily calorie requirements

Measuring body fat

The most common and unintrusive way to measure body fat is by using a Bio-electrical Impedance Analysis (BIA) Machine. A BIA body fat scale measures the resistance of a mild electrical current as it flows between electrodes attached to two specific points of the body, either the hand and opposite foot or from one foot to another. Body fat creates a greater resistance whereas lean tissue is a good conductor of electricity. The result is an indicator of body composition although it can overestimate lean tissue of muscular people or underestimate body fat of overweight people by 2–3 per cent.

The other most available method is that of skin fold measurements by using callipers that measure the millimetres of fat just underneath the skin. The accuracy of this method depends on the person who is taking the measurements and also assumes that fat distribution is the same for everyone as they age. According to Houtkooper (2000) and Lohman (1992), the estimated margin of error for skin fold measurements is 3-4 per cent. Therefore a body fat measurement of 25 per cent could actually be anywhere between 21–22 per cent or 28–29 per cent.

Working out basal metabolic rate

There are several formulas for working out BMR, and you are likely to already be using a tried and tested method. However, I have included the following Katch–McArdle formula as it takes into account body composition, and can be applied to both men and women:

BMR formula for men and women = 370 + (21.6 x lean mass in Kg)

Example:
Male: age 60
Weight: 75 kg
Body fat: 22 per cent (16.5 kg)
Lean Mass: 68 per cent (58.5 kg)
BMR = 370 + (21.6 x 58.5) = 1,634 calories
less 8 per cent (2 per cent per decade over age 20) = 131 calories
1,634 – 131 = 1,503
BMR = 1,503.

This is the total number of calories required for essential body functions *excluding* calories used for daily activity and exercise.

Mostly sedentary, seated or standing activities during the day	BMR x 1.4
Moderately active – regular brisk walking or equivalent during the day	BMR x 1.7
Very active on a daily basis and takes physical exercise	BMR x 2.0

Adding on exercise and activity calories

Source - The Complete Guide to Sports Nutrition (4th edition), Anita Bean (2003)

These calculations for working out correct calorie intake are guidelines to help your client lose or maintain weight. Calorie intake should never be lower than the BMR as this could lead to the loss of important calorie-burning muscle tissue.

Changes to the cardiovascular system

General changes to the cardiovascular system include a loss of size and strength to the muscle

Figure 2.2 Cardiovascular system

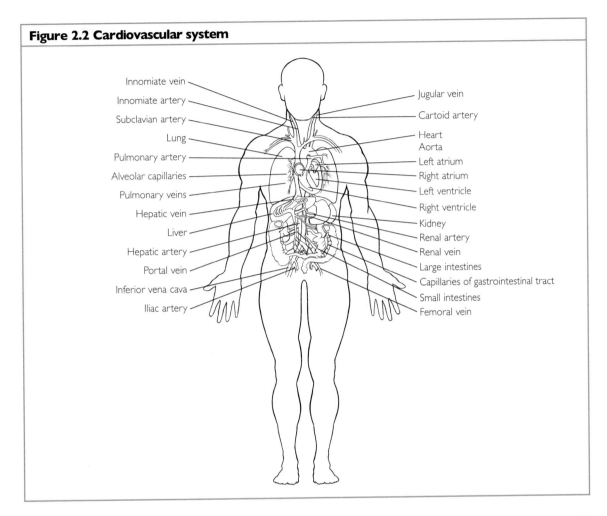

in the wall of the heart (cardiac muscle). This causes a reduction in the volume of oxygenated blood flow from the heart (cardiac output), a reduction in the maximum heart rate and an increase in systolic blood pressure.

The ageing process causes a progressive decline in VO_2 max that can be linked to the tendency of people to become more sedentary after the age of 30. Maximal aerobic capacity decreases in both men and woman with an average decline of about 10 per cent per decade between the ages of 25–65 (Hawkins, Marcell, Jaque and Wiswell, 2001). The decline occurs

slowly at first and then becomes more rapid, particularly in sedentary people, and the long-term or accumulative effect of inactivity begins to show after the age of 60.

Another change to the cardiovascular system that affects aerobic capacity is the amount of blood that leaves the heart per minute of peak exercise:

- **maximal cardiac output** decreases by 1 per cent per year between the age of 35 and 65 (Helloszy, 2001) and blood flow to the muscles is reduced (Ho, Beard, Farrell, Miason & Kenney, 1997).

- **maximal heart rate (MHR)** reduces by 5–10 beats per minute per decade (Wiebe, Gledhill, Jammik & Ferguson, 1999).
- **maximal stroke volume** (the volume of blood pumped with each heartbeat) is also reduced (Proctor, Beck *et al.*, 1999).

Blood Cholesterol

As people age it is important to keep blood cholesterol under control as it increases the risk of heart disease. The body needs cholesterol to digest fat, make hormones and build cells, and it is carried in the blood in particles called lipoproteins, which deliver the cholesterol to the various body tissues. There are two types of blood cholesterol; low-density lipoproteins (LDL) and high-density lipoproteins (HDL):

1. too much LDL (also referred to as 'damaging cholesterol') will cause a build up of harmful fatty or plaque in the arteries. If there is too much LDL circulating, arteries will be damaged and impede blood to the heart, leading to the heart muscle being starved of oxygen. If an artery is completely blocked by plaque this can lead to a heart attack.
2. HDL (considered 'protective' cholesterol) helps prevent a build up and carries blood cholesterol back to the liver so that waste can be eliminated from the body. Low HDL will also increase the risk of heart disease.

When cholesterol levels are checked the blood is checked for another type of blood fat called triglycerides which, if too high, are an additional risk of heart disease. High LDL increases the risk of coronary heart disease, as narrowed arteries cannot transport enough blood to the heart muscle during exertion. This results in a lack of oxygen in the heart muscle, and causes chest pain.

The benefits of exercise on blood cholesterol

- reduced LDL
- reduced triglycerides
- increased HDL

The effects of these physical changes during exercise means that there is much more strain on the heart, leading to a reduced blood supply to working muscles, causing inactive and older people to get tired much faster. Maximal oxygen intake is affected by previous activity levels, so for individuals that have participated in regular long-term aerobic training, the rate at which VO_2 max declines is slower, although MHR still reduces by 5–10 beats per minute per decade.

Although the rate of decline of aerobic capacity in older adults can be slowed down, it can't be stopped entirely. However, it is very important to let your clients know that much of the ageing process is within their control, and that participating in regular physical activity can delay the normal ageing process by 10–20 years (Shepard, 1997).

The implications of cardiovascular (CV) changes on exercise

When designing the aerobic component of an exercise programme, or an exercise to music class, remember that the aerobic capacity requirement is much less for older adults, and the goal tends to be more about retaining function and achieving a sense of wellbeing. This does, however, depend on the history of your client and what their personal goals are. For general programme and class design, build in longer warm up and cool down periods. A warm up should be 15 minutes of lower intensity exercise that will give the CV system time to safely adjust to the extra exertion. A longer cool down of 10 minutes is also required to prevent venous pooling in the legs that can lead to rapid drops in blood pressure and light-headedness or fainting after exercise. A gradual cool down will also prevent the chances of post exercise cardiac rhythm disturbances, arrhythmias (changes in rhythm of the heart beat), that can be brought on by high levels of circulating exercise hormones.

The benefits of exercise on the cardiovascular system

- increased calorie expenditure during exercise and at rest
- improved efficiency of the heart muscle (myocardial performance)
- increased diastolic filling (which refers to the volume and efficiency of pumping blood through the heart)
- increased heart muscle contractility (when beats per minute are at a constant rate)
- improved blood lipid profile – a blood test that measures total cholesterol, HDL and LDL and triglycerides to assess risk of heart disease (see blood cholesterol on page 14).
- reduced systolic blood pressure (the pressure on the artery walls during the contraction and relaxation of the heart)
- improved diastolic blood pressure (the force of blood against the artery walls in between heart contractions)
- improved endurance
- improved muscle capillary blood flow, which improves the flow of oxygenated blood to the working muscles.

Monitoring heart rate

Maximal Heart Rate (HR max) decreases by as much as 10 beats per minute per decade from its peak at the age of 20. However, using the HR max formula is not the best way to determine the correct intensity for older clients. In a study by Paterson and colleagues in 1999, they found that HR max = 220 – age underestimated the actual measured HR max in men by 6–11 beats, and in women by 7–9 beats, per minute.

The effects of medication such as beta-blockers that are commonly described for high blood pressure and cardiac conditions can reduce resting heart rate by as much as 30 beats per minute. The safest way for you and your client to measure heart rate or beats per minute (bpm) is by using Borg's Rate of Perceived Exertion scale (see page 34).

Blood pressure

There is a progressive rise in resting and exercise blood pressure as we age (Franklin, 2000) which elevates the heart's work rate and oxygen needs. While both systolic and diastolic blood pressure increases with age, several studies have shown that physical activity can reduce systolic and diastolic blood pressure in patients with borderline hypertension. (Hagberg & Goldberg, 1990). Physical activity has both long and short term effects on blood pressure. In the long term, physical activity may reduce blood pressure by preventing obesity, reducing insulin dependence and increasing the density of muscle, and in the short term immediately after exercise there are changes in the mechanisms that regulate and determine blood pressure.

Changes to the respiratory system

The cardiovascular system and the respiratory system work together, and if either system is damaged or diseased it will affect the other.

The decline in the efficiency of the pulmonary system is due to a combination of changes. The reduced strength of the respiratory muscle, increased stiffness of the chest wall and closure of small arteries makes breathing more difficult. The connective tissue in the lungs also loses elasticity and reduces the efficiency of gaseous exchange during exercise. As we age, there are changes to the anatomy and physiology of the thorax, which reduces the capacity and efficiency of the lungs to absorb and transport oxygen:

- the rib cage becomes more rigid and loses its elasticity
- poor or stooped posture (kyphosis) reduces chest capacity

Figure 2.3 Respiratory system

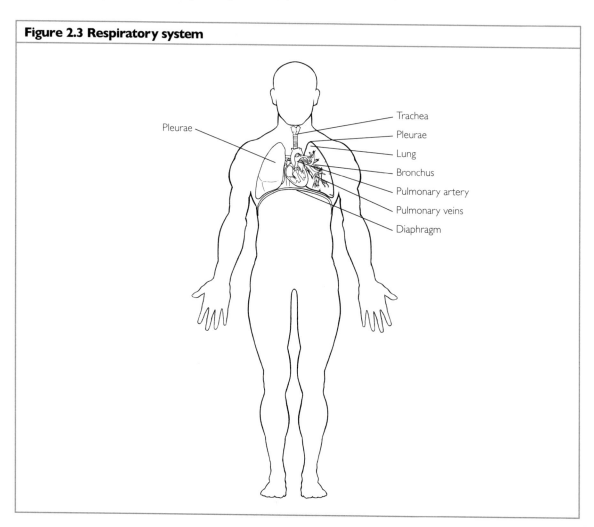

Pleurae

Trachea
Pleurae
Lung
Bronchus
Pulmonary artery
Pulmonary veins
Diaphragm

- lack of use because of a sedentary lifestyle will also result in poor respiratory function
- the tissues in the lungs and bronchi become less elastic and affect the breathing movement and flow.

The efficiency of the lungs, and the maximum air that a person can exhale after a full inhalation, decreases by up to 40–50 per cent by the age of 70:

- Gaseous exchange steadily declines with age.
- Between the ages of 30 and 70 the maximum air breathed in per minute (maximal voluntary ventilation) reduces by up to 50 per cent.
- The amount of air remaining in the lungs after breathing out (residual lung volume) increases by 30–50 per cent (Daley & Spinks, 2000).

However, moderate to high intensity physical activity may prevent age related decline in resting lung function until the age of 60 (Pollock *et al.*, 1997).

The implications of respiratory system changes on exercise

Pulmonary gas exchange does not usually limit exercise ability in older adults unless they have a chronic condition such as coronary heart disease (CHD) or chronic obstructive pulmonary disorder (COPD) (see Part 3). However, older adults have less tolerance for shortness of breath – it can make them feel anxious and they will be more likely to stop exercising from fear of overexerting themselves. If there is not enough oxygen the body will produce the energy it needs anaerobically. This will lead to a build up in lactic acid, and the resulting discomfort from muscle soreness can put your client off their exercise programme.

> An exercise programme that includes diaphragmatic breathing that increases elasticity in the thoracic cage (see Part 3), as well as Yoga, Tai Chi and Pilates, will improve breathing technique and build the confidence of your older client.

Muscular changes

There is a gradual loss of skeletal muscle from around the age of 30, which may be partly attributed to a sedentary lifestyle. Age related changes in muscle function are:

- decreased muscle strength
- decreased muscle power
- decreased muscle endurance
- decreased muscle mass (sarcopeneia)
- reduction in the number of motor units that stimulate muscle fibres so that they can contract.

A brief revision of muscle fibre types may help here: Muscle is made up of two types of fibre, type I and type II.

- type I are slow twitch (ST) and slow to fatigue
- type II are fast twitch (FT) and quick to fatigue.

Research has shown that slow twitch fibres show little change in older people (Thompson, 2002), whereas fast twitch fibres decrease between 25–50 per cent in the number of, and size of, muscle fibres between the ages of 20 and 80 years.

There are high numbers of fast twitch fibres in the back, buttocks, quadriceps, hamstrings and calves, which are essential for leg strength and balance. These are the first to atrophy in older adults because of a lack of high intensity activity that is required to activate fast twitch fibres (Landers, Hunter, Wetzstein, Barnam & Wiensier, 2001).

Figure 2.4 Muscles of the body

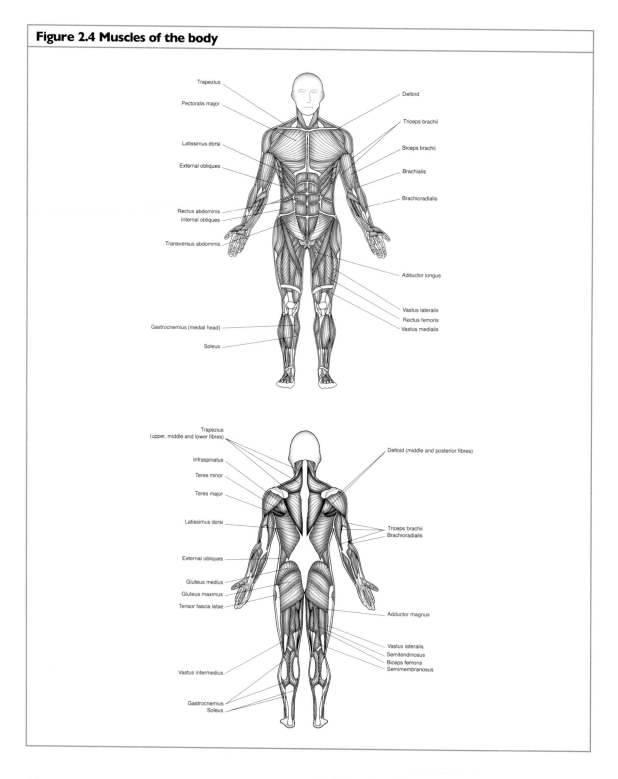

Muscle strength

Muscle strength decreases by approximately 30 per cent between the ages of 50 and 70. As with muscle mass there is a greater loss in the lower body due in part to inactivity as well as the reduction of motor neurons.

Muscle power

Muscle power diminishes to an even greater extent than muscle strength (Foldvari *et al.,* 2000), and is caused by inactivity, atrophy of fast twitch fibres and a decrease in motor units. These all combine and result in a loss of the ability to move quickly against a force (Krivikas *et al.,* 2001). For example, walking up stairs, rising from seating to standing or recovering from tripping.

Changes in mitochondria

According to Robert Robergs, an exercise physiologist at the University for New Mexico, a good training programme can *double* mitochondria mass in the muscles that do the work. He suggests at least 30 minutes of sustained jogging, swimming, cycling or walking at a moderate to high intensity every day.

Mitochondria is responsible for energy production in the cycle of converting ATP (Andenosine triphosphate) to ADP (Andenosine diphosphate) and back to ATP, which coverts glucose into energy. In other words, mitochondria is the powerhouse that leads the way in converting carbohydrates, protein, fat and alcohol into fuel for the muscles while we work and rest.

Researchers have found that as we get older mitochondria slowly self destructs, and studies have shown that mitochondrial decay can cause a number of disorders associated with ageing, such as Alzheimer's disease, obesity, diabetes, and ageing itself. According to Douglas Wallace, a geneticist at the University of California, mitochondria can cause harm through the same process in which it converts oxygen, fat and carbohydrates to produce energy for activity. During the process of catabolism (breaking down molecules of nutrients), there are damaging oxygen radicals produced which can injure protein lipids and DNA and damage mitochondria. Over time, damaged mitochondria begin to falter and produce less energy and will eventually die.

Howard Hughes and Gerald Shulmans of Yale University School of Medicine have studied the number and function of mitochondria of different age groups. They found that a lean, healthy 70 year old has more fat in their muscle and liver cells, has half the number of mitochondria and does not burn as many calories as a 20 year old of the same condition and weight.

Implications of muscle changes on exercise

Exercise programmes for older adults should focus on promoting *hypertrophy* – increasing mass fast twitch fibres – particularly in the back, buttocks, thighs and calves. Many of the age related changes of muscle function could be minimised or even reversed. Resistance training can reduce or prevent decline in muscle function and is considered to be important for preventing muscle atrophy, muscle weakness and loss of muscle power (Roth *et al.,* 2000). Resistance training will also improve bone health, improve postural stability that will reduce the risk of falls, increase calorie expenditure, decrease body fat mass and increase flexibility and range of movement in older adults.

According to Robert Robergs, an exercise physiologist at the University for New Mexico, a good training programme can double mitochondria mass in the muscles that do the work, and suggests at least 30 minutes of **sustained** jogging, swimming, cycling or walking at a moderate to high intensity every day.

Aerobic endurance training will also improve the aerobic function of muscles, their ability to utilise oxygen, and can minimise many age related changes in muscular mass, muscle strength and muscle power.

When designing your programme be aware of your clients' physiological limitations of utilising their energy stores and the capacity of their reduced muscle strength and endurance. The initial level at which you begin to develop, or enhance, your clients' fitness level should keep them within their comfort zone.

Changes in flexibility

There are significant changes in flexibility as we age – joints become stiffer and unstable. This is partly due to age related changes in the elasticity of connective tissue and the stiffening or shortening of the ligaments, tendons, joint capsules, muscles, fascia and skin around the joint that reduces joint mobility. Synovial fluid that lubricates the joint also decreases and cartilage and bone can begin to rub and cause pain and discomfort in the joints.

Flexibility is also reduced through lack of use and inactivity. Research has shown flexibility declines 20–50 percent between the ages of 30 and 70 years (Fatouras *et al.*, 2002). The effects this has on range of motion (ROM) can lead to problems in an individual's ability to perform daily tasks such as climbing stairs, dressing and getting into the car. A lack of flexibility also increases the risk of injury to the muscles crossing the joint and causes greater instability and loss of balance, increasing the risk of a fall.

Implications of changes in flexibility on exercise

Not all older people lose flexibility at the same rate, and active older adults show more flexibility in the hips, spine, ankles and knees than those who are inactive (Daly & Spinks, 2000). All exercise programmes and classes need to include stretching and mobility exercise. Static and dynamic stretching have shown to increase range of movement (ROM) in older adults, although the training effect is joint specific (Barbesa *et al.*, 2002).

Skeletal changes

There are two key changes in bone tissue as people age:

1. a loss of calcium and bone mineral
2. a decrease in the rate of protein synthesis, decreasing the body's ability to produce collagen which gives bone its tensile strength (tension and stretch). This is why bones become more brittle and susceptible to fracture.

Changes in bone density

Bone Mineral Density (BMD) refers to the ratio of deposited mineral salts to organic bone. A loss or reduction of BMD can result in osteoporosis (See Part Three for more information on this). BMD peaks at around the age of 25 (Marcus, 2001) and remains stable until around the age of 50, after which a gradual loss of calcium and deterioration of bone occurs in both men and women. There is a much more rapid loss of calcium in women during the five years after menopause (Drinkwater, 1994), and women are three times more likely to develop osteoporosis that men.

Figure 2.5 Human skeleton

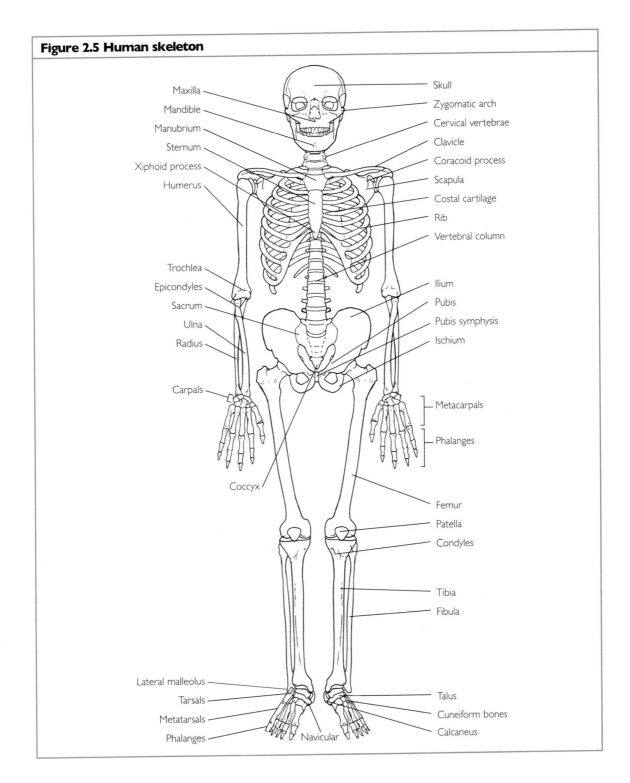

Implications for changes in bone density on exercise

Osteoporosis and exercise is covered fully in Part Three, and other general considerations are as follows. As there is an increased risk of fracture, it is important to give consideration to how you can minimise the risk of your client falling in both the exercise environment you provide and in the exercise you recommend. Be aware of blind steps in the gym or mat corners that stick up or any stray hand weights or loose equipment that could be a health and safety risk. It is also important to be aware that an osteoporatic spine is very vulnerable, so avoid exercise that involves spinal flexion (bending forward), twisting and sudden movements.

There has been much investigation into the effects of physical activity on BMD, and there is evidence that the right programme may prevent or reverse bone loss at the lumber spine and femoral neck (hip) of pre- and post-menopausal woman by almost 1 per cent per year (Blanchet *et al.*, 2002). Research has also shown that the intensity of exercise is more important on BMD than frequency (Vincent & Braithwaite, 2002). Heavier weights and fewer repetitions result in greater gains in bone mass than lighter loads with higher repetitions (Metcalfe *et al.*, 2001). Weight bearing exercises such as walking, jogging and stair climbing have shown to be more effective for building bone in the hip than those that create stress through joint action (for example weight lifting and rowing). Other studies have shown that the leg press, overhead press and lumbar extension exercises have the greatest influence on specific joint and total body BMD (Vincent and Braithwaite, 2002).

Intervertebral discs and spine

The intervertebral discs are soft pads of cartilage that sit between the vertebrae. Their purpose is to hold the vertebrae of the spine together, act as a shock absorber to carry the downward weight of the body (axial load) when we are standing, and they also act as a pivot point, which allows the spine to bend and twist. As we age, discs thin and lose fluid. This results in the spine becoming more curved and compressed and is noticeable by the reduced length in the trunk.

Benefits of physical activity on musculoskeletal system

- reduced risk of musculoskeletal disability
- improved strength and flexibility
- reduced risk of falls
- improved dynamic balance
- improved physical function
- slower decline in bone mineral density
- increased total body calcium.

Changes in the nervous system

The nervous system has two parts:

1. the **central nervous system** which consists of the brain and the spinal cord
2. the **peripheral nervous system** which consists of the nerves that travel to and from the spine, carrying messages to the central nervous system.

As we age, the number of nerve cells (neurons) decreases, which causes atrophy to the brain and the spinal cord. These cells reduce in size and the branches that carry messages are also reduced, which slows down the speed at which the message is sent. After a message has been

Figure 2.6 Central and peripheral nervous system

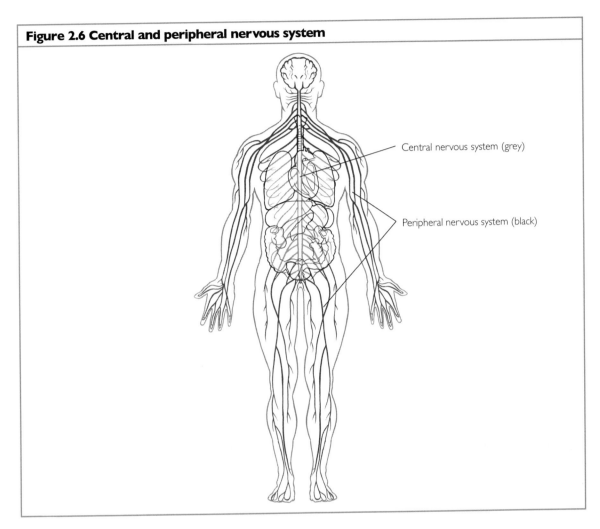

Central nervous system (grey)

Peripheral nervous system (black)

sent there is a rest period before another message can be sent, called the latency period. Ageing increases the length of the rest period between thoughts, and therefore thinking and response time will be slower. This does *not* mean that all older people will develop illnesses such as Alzheimer's or senile dementia, but that individuals will need more time to process information as they get older. Degeneration and disease of nerve cells can also affect vision, hearing and touch, all of which will affect balance and increase the risk of falls.

Cognition

The changes in the mental process of ageing do not affect everyone in the same way. Generally, older adults develop memory loss after the age of 70. However, research has shown that physical activity and improved fitness have a beneficial effect on memory and other cognitive processes (Etruer & Berg, 2001; Laurin, Verrealt, Lindsay, Macpherson & Rockwood, 2001; Yaffe, Barnes, Nevin, Lai & Corvinski, 2001).

Implications of cognitive changes on exercise

As we age there is a gradual decline in the cognitive efficiency of memory, both short- and long-term, attention span, intelligence and the speed at which information can be absorbed and processed. According to Silverstone (2001), steady declines are evident from the age of 30. It becomes gradually more difficult to divide attention between tasks (for example, listening to an instruction while concentrating on a particular movement or carrying out an exercise), and speed of thought and reaction time is slower. For example, an older client who is intensely focused on a move in an exercise class, or the action of exercise equipment, will stop what they are doing if somebody speaks to them or asks them a question. Your older clients will also take longer to respond to your instruction, especially if it is new information. Keep information clear and specific, and make sure that it relates to their specific goals and needs.

Make sure that your exercise area is well lit. Older adults need four times more light that younger people.

Psychological benefits of exercise

1. Improves perceived wellbeing and happiness
2. Decreases levels of stress related hormones
3. Improves attention span
4. Improves cognitive processing speed

Changes in the sensory and motor systems

As people age you may well have observed that, to differing degrees, their reactions and response times become slower, movements may appear to be slightly awkward and gait or step while walking seems to widen sideways, indicating a degree of instability. This is a result of *somatosensory* changes – the awareness of the body's parts in relation to each other and the orientation of the body in space and touch sensitivity. The three main sources of sensory information that influence these changes are:

1. **Proprioceptive information** from the muscles and joints, which tells the brain the position of the limbs and their movements. The signals from the receptors in the joints, ligaments, tendons and muscles indicate when to change position or adapt a movement (for example, on the approach to a step up or a step down).
2. **Vestibular information** from the canals in the inner ear helps to orientate the body in space while resting or moving. The canals are filled with fluid, granules and sensitive hairs that react to gravity and provide information to the brain regarding the movement, direction and speed of the head (see figure 2.7 below).
3. **Visual information** from the eyes. There is 'reduced visual acuity' (the ability to see objects clearly), an increase in eye disease and a greater likelihood of poor eyesight in older people. There may be an increased sensitivity to glare and poor depth perception that can lead to poor judgement of ground surfaces or distance, making older adults more vulnerable to trips and falls. Be aware of the following changes that can be expected in older adults so that you can adapt your exercise programme

Figure 2.7 Inside the ear

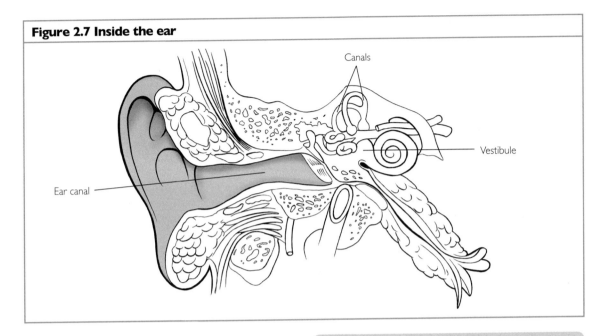

Canals

Vestibule

Ear canal

and be alert to environmental conditions that might make it difficult for your client to see clearly (see figure 2.8 below).

Both hearing and vision decline with age. Background noise can be particularly frustrating for older adults who have lost their ability to mask our surrounding sound which impairs their ability to take instruction, and they may feel too embarrassed to say anything.

Figure 2.8 Common eye conditions in older adults

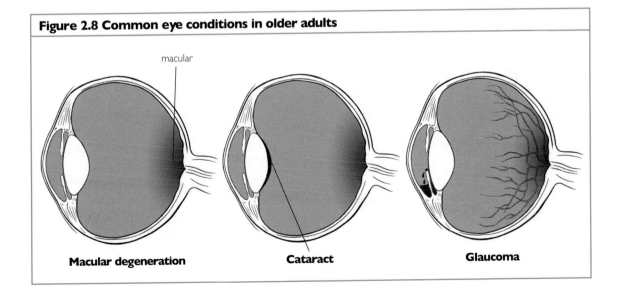

macular

Macular degeneration   **Cataract**   **Glaucoma**

Table 2.1	Changes to the eyes	
Common eye conditions	Effects	Exercise and environment considerations
Presbyopia	Reduced ability to see close objects or small print. Symptoms include holding reading materials at arms length and headaches or tired eyes when reading.	Programme cards written clearly with bold lettering. Check that your client can see the control panels and buttons of gym equipment clearly.
Corneal disease and related conditions Retinal Disorders	A **cataract** makes it difficult to let light pass through the lens and can cause loss of eyesight. **Glaucoma** is caused by increased fluid pressure inside the eye, which can, over time, lead to vision loss and blindness. **Age related macular degeneration (AMD)** affects the retina (the macula), and causes a decline in the sharp central vision needed to see objects and read clearly. **Diabetic retinopathy** happens when small blood vessels stop feeding from the retina. **Retinal detachment** happens when the inner and outer layers of the retina separate. This condition requires surgery or laser treatment.	Can cause reduced or blurred vision. Be aware of obstacles such as steps or mat corners that can easily be missed and free weights left on the floor. Be aware of any awkwardly positioned equipment that could be a hazard to a client with poor vision. Check that your client is able to hold on for support while getting off the equipment. Check there is enough space between machines for your clients to move safely.
Floaters	These are tiny specks or flecks that seem to float across the eyes, and are very common. They do not in themselves cause a problem, although they might be an indication of a more serious problem if they are accompanied with light flashes. If this is the case they will need medical attention.	

Table 2.1	Changes to the eyes *cont.*	
Common eye conditions	Effects	Exercise and environment considerations
Dry Eyes	Caused by tear glands not producing enough fluid, resulting in itching or burning, and may cause some loss of vision.	As above
Luminance	The amount of light that reaches the back of the eye decreases and older people get less light through a smaller pupil.	Make sure the area you are working in is well lit. On average, older adults require four times more light than younger people.
Sensitivity to glare	Bright light that shines directly or reflects into the eye can make it difficult to focus. Older people's ability to recover from glare or bright lights decreases after age 50 due to changes in the lens of the eye.	Be aware of how light reflects off the equipment, especially from shiny surfaces and control panels.
Light/dark adaptation	As people age there are changes to pupil size, affecting the amount of light reaching the retina. This is accompanied by a thickening of the lens, which makes it difficult to adapt to changes in lighting conditions.	Eyes need time to adapt if lighting conditions change.
Light/dark contrast	As people age they need increasingly sharper contrasts and sharper edges around an object to differentiate it from its background. The ability to distinguish colours that are similar in hue such as blue and green or red and orange also becomes more difficult.	Older people need high contrast printed materials such as sharp, crisp black lettering on white background. Be aware of font size and colours on posters and programme cards – they should preferably be at least 12 or 14 point size.
Reduced depth perception	It becomes more difficult to judge how near or far away or how high or low something is.	Highlight steps and slopes to your client and make sure these areas are well lit without glare.

Information from the senses is received by the brain for central processing, and channelled to the relevant part to help maintain balance and equilibrium. Any deterioration or age related slowing down of this central processing puts older adults at greater risk of falls and they are more likely to make mistakes or trip and lose their balance when they move quickly. Emphasis during instruction of exercise needs to focus on *accuracy* of technique at a *slower pace* and gradually build up speed over time.

Fortunately, balance can be improved because the sensory systems are very adaptable. An essential component of a programme or class for the older adult should be at least 10–15 minutes of balance and mobility exercises. These should challenge your client without going beyond their capabilities. A gradual progression in the degree of difficulty will build confidence and keep them motivated.

The studio and gym should be well lit, and be aware of the noise level, in particular how loud the music is. As the instructor of older adults you will increase your skills as an instructor and put your older clients at ease if you have a bank of visual clues, signals and body language that you can employ to help your client understand your instruction more clearly. You would also benefit from learning to read your clients' body language and signals. Frequently check their understanding and become sensitive to their reaction, ask yourself how comfortable they look. Are they giving you their full attention? Is something distracting them?

Careful observation and showing empathy

Specific balance training and core stability group classes such as Tai Chi, Yoga, and Pilates can be easily adapted to suit the level of your older adult. The use of stability balls and foam-based mats provide a suitable and challenging base while performing upper body exercises.

for your clients will prevent them from the embarrassment of asking you to repeat yourself and will ensure their health and safety during their training session.

References

Egger, G. and Champion, N. (1990) *The Fitness Leaders Handbook*, third edition (A&C Black)

Jessie Jones, C. and Rose, Debra J. (2005), *Physical Activity Instruction of Older Adults* (Human Kinetics)

Oxford Concise Medical Dictionary (2003, Oxford University Press)

Tortora, G. J. and Grabowski, S. R. (1993) *Principles of Anatomy and Physiology*, seventh edition (HarperCollins)

Online resources

www.bpassoc.org.uk, the Blood Pressure Association.

www.nice.org.uk, NICE is the independent organisation responsible for providing national guidance on the promotion of good health and the prevention and treatment of ill health.

Table 2.2	Summary of physiological changes of ageing	
Cardiovascular system	**Age change occurs**	**Description of change**
VO$_2$ max	25–65	Maximal oxygen consumption or total oxygen that can be utilised by the muscles decreases by about 10 per cent per decade or 1 per cent per year.
Maximal cardiac output	35–65	The amount of blood pumped by the heart each minute also decreases by 10 per cent per decade or 1 per cent per year and also reduces the amount of blood flow to the muscles.
Maximal stroke volume		The amount of blood that is pumped by the heart in each beat decreases with age.
Maximal heart rate		The highest heart rate a person can attain during exercise reduces by 5-10 beats per decade.
Blood pressure		There is a progressive increase in systolic and diastolic in resting and exercise blood pressure as people age. 140/90 mmHg is the start of high BP and medication may be required for BP readings of 160/100 mmHg.
Pulmonary system		
Maximal voluntary ventilation	By the age of 70	Air breathed in per minute decreases by 50 per cent by the age of 70.
Maximal alveolar ventilation		The maximum amount of air exchanged between the atmosphere and the alveoli in the lungs is reduced during exercise in older adults.
Residual lung volume		The amount of air remaining in the lungs increases by up to 30-50 per cent.
Musculoskeletal system		
Muscle strength	50–70	Muscle strength decreases by approximately 30 per cent due in part to inactivity.
Muscle power		Muscle power decreases because of inactivity and muscle atrophy.
Type II muscle fibres		Type II fast contracting muscle fibres decrease 20-50 per cent in quantity and size.
Flexibility	30–70	Flexibility decreases 20-50 per cent.
Bone mineral density	50+	There is a gradual loss of bone mineral density for both men and women and a more rapid loss for women during the five years after menopause.
Cognitive function		There can be a gradual decline in short and long term memory, speed and thought and reaction time can be slower and dividing attention between tasks can be more difficult. Changes in cognitive, sensory and motor systems will affect balance, stability and co-ordination.
Vision and hearing		Reduced visual acuity (the ability to see objects clearly), increased sensitivity to glare, poor depth perception and changes in the structure of the ear that affect hearing and balance.

NB: The above summary does give a rather bleak view of the ageing process, and although there are inevitable changes associated with ageing, the good news is that research has shown that much of the ageing process is within our control, and that the normal ageing process can be delayed by 10–20 years.

THE PRINCIPLES OF FITNESS
FOR OLDER ADULTS

PART **TWO**

INSTRUCTING OLDER ADULTS

3

The older population consists of a diverse range of fitness levels and abilities. There are many older adults who compete as master athletes, as well as those who have problems getting out of a chair. A programme for an older adult needs to be individually tailored to their specific health and fitness levels, with consideration given to their previous exercise experience, their personal goals and any chronic conditions they might have.

Many older adults are highly likely to have one or more chronic conditions (specific chronic conditions are covered in detail in Part Three) that will put some limitation on their physical functioning, although many older adults have no chronic conditions. As an instructor you can help your clients to maintain their physical functioning, and also rise to the challenge of creating exercise programmes that accommodate the diverse health conditions and physical abilities of older clients.

Functional fitness is the primary motivation for the majority of older adults, whereas mid-life adults may be more focused on preventing decline and the onset of age related diseases. If you can spend time explaining the functional and preventative benefits of being active it will give your client's programme more personal relevance and meaning. A key motivator for adults is retaining mobility and independence for as long as possible.

The American College of Sports Medicine (ACSM) guidelines for Exercise Testing and Prescription (ACSM, 2000) recommend that older adults accumulate at least 30 minutes of moderate intensity exercise on most days, and preferably all days, of the week. Resistance training of at least 2 sessions per week on alternate days and flexibility training of at least 2–3 sessions per week is recommended to maintain flexibility, agility and balance.

The principles of fitness for older adults

The principles of *overload* and *specificity* remain the same, and there are three more specifically for the older adult that have been introduced by experts in Geronkinesiology (see below). They are *functional relevance, challenge* and *accommodation.*

The principle of overload

This principle states that an individual must exercise at a level above that which can normally be carried out comfortably. The intensity duration and frequency of the exercise should be greater than they are normally accustomed to and will result in an adaptation that can lead to improved physical function. With some knowledge of the physiological changes that occur with age you would expect progress to be slower for older adults.

Table 3.1	Guidelines for applying overload principles
Increase only one variable at a time (speed or load or repetition or time or frequency)	
Increase duration before intensity	
Increase duration in one minute increments as tolerated (Fiatarone, Singh, 2000)	
Increase intensity by using arms (e.g. arms above the waist) or by increasing the speed of movement (Singh, 2000)	
Allow a minimum of two weeks for adaptation before increasing overload (Dinan, 2002)	

Extracted from *Physical Activity Instruction of Older Adults* by Jones and Rose (2005)

The principle of specificity

This principle states that the training effects of physical activity are specific to the types of exercise and muscles involved (ACSM, 2000). For example, the exercises selected for aerobic endurance must be specific to the energy systems being targeted, aerobic or anaerobic (Bompa, 1999). If you apply this to lifestyle, your programme could also provide exercises that will develop your clients' ability to respond to sudden bursts of energy that might be required in daily living and leisure activities, for example going up stairs or walking up a hill.

The principle of functional relevance

This principle refers to how an exercise programme reflects the movements required in daily living. For example, balance and mobility training could include carrying out exercises on surfaces that are more challenging, such as foam or a stability ball. The principle of functional relevance adds to the motivation of your clients because it emphasises the relevance of exercise to their everyday life, and gives more purpose and meaning to the effort required. Functional relevance exercises for aerobic endurance include stair climbing and descending, and picking up objects. Including specific functional tasks in your programme will improve muscle strength and functional ability (Skelton & McLaughlin, 1996).

The principle of challenge

This principle differs from the principle of overload as it emphasises the importance of staying within the capabilities of your client. It is important to identify the point at which your client is challenged enough to achieve a training effect without putting them at risk of injury or causing them discomfort. You may find that some clients are keen to push themselves on quickly and you may need all your skills of diplomacy to persuade them to progress more slowly. There will be others who will be more fearful and will need encouragement to push beyond their boundaries, but only a little and within a safe range. Adding a task, for example bringing in arm movements while moving across the room, can increase the challenge of aerobic endurance exercises.

The principle of accommodation

This principle advises that your participants should be encouraged to perform exercises to the best of their ability, but that they should never push themselves to a point of pain, over exertion or beyond a level they consider to be safe (Jones, 2001). This principle is applied to older adults who have chronic conditions and functional weaknesses, and encourages them to go at their own preferred pace and to the best of their ability. If your client is taking medication for one or more medical conditions, it is important to recognise that there may be days when it will affect their ability to exercise, and the intensity at which they can exercise. Conditions such as arthritis can 'flare up' and you will need to both provide exercise adaptations and teach your client to monitor their exertion and level of pain (see Part Three for more information on chronic conditions).

THE COMPONENTS OF AN EXERCISE PROGRAMME FOR OLDER ADULTS

4

The warm up

A physiological definition of warming up is increasing the temperature of muscles and blood in preparation for the body's transition from rest to activity (Nieman, 1999). The age related changes to the cardiovascular, musculoskeletal and neuromuscular systems put even greater emphasis on the need to prepare thoroughly for activity. The slower reaction times, loss of elasticity, strength and aerobic capacity also indicate that we need to encourage older clients to spend more time warming up, and progress slowly to more vigorous activity. Warming up increases the blood saturation to all systems, improves delivery of oxygen to the cells and increases elasticity of muscles, tendons and joints. Improved elasticity is particularly important for injury prevention in older adults.

The transition from small to larger ranges of movement needs to be gradual, allowing the mind and the body to adapt for what is to come. Teach your clients the Borg's RPE scale (see table 4.1), and monitor their responses with a talk test – your client should be able to respond with a sentence to a question without gasping for breath. Advise your clients to keep the level of intensity on Borg's 6–20 scale between 9–10 and for frailer or more sedentary adults between 7–9. The warm up should be at least 15 minutes in length and frailer or more sedentary clients may require a longer warm up of 20 minutes.

Table 4.1	Borg's rating of perceived exertion	
Number	Effort level	Perceived exertion
6	20%	Very, very light
7	30%	
8	40%	
9	50%	Very light
10	55%	
11	60%	Fairly light
12	65%	
13	70%	Moderately hard
14	75%	
15	80%	Hard
16	85%	
17	90%	Very hard
18	95%	
19	100%	Very, very hard
20		Exhaustion

Recommendations for levels of intensity for older adults

RPE Scale Instructions

During the exercise test we want you to pay close attention to how hard you feel the exercise work rate is.

The feeling should reflect your total amount of exertion and fatigue, combining all sensations and feelings of physical stress, effort and fatigue.

Don't concern yourself with any one factor such as leg pain, shortness of breath or exercise intensity, but try to concentrate on your total, inner feeling of exertion. Try not to underestimate or overestimate your feelings of exertion, be as accurate as you can.

Instructions as recommended by ACSM, 2002 p.79

RPE scale guidance

The RPE Scale instructions recommended for clients are as follows:

- a training intensity between 13–15 on the 6–20 RPE scale is approximately equivalent to working at 70–80 per cent of VO_2 max. An RPE of 11–13 is approximately 49–70 per cent of VO_2 max (ACSM, 1990).
- the guideline for the starting point for sedentary older adults is an RPE of 11–13 (light to somewhat hard) and should **not** exceed an RPE of 15 (hard) (ACSM, 1990).
- for frailer older adults the recommendation is to begin at an RPE of 9–11 (very light to light).

Be aware of room temperature. According to the ACSM, an ambient room temperature is unsafe if it exceeds 82° F (28° C) for vigorous exercise or 84° F (29° C) for moderate exercise.

The cool down

A cool down of at least ten minutes is as essential as the warm up. The cool down phase should reduce body temperature, heart rate and respiration, gradually bringing them back to pre–activity levels. Mild continuous activity following exercise keeps the leg muscles contracting and will promote venous return (blood flowing to the heart). This will prevent the blood from pooling in the extremities, and reduces the likelihood of the dizziness and fainting that can happen if exercise suddenly stops. A low intensity cool down will also speed up the removal of lactic acid in the muscles and blood, and speed up recovery.

A cool down helps to decrease the level of *catecholamines* (adrenaline and noradrenaline), that are both neurotransmitters, and hormones which are raised during exercise. High levels of catecholamines can cause cardiac irregularities usually after, rather than during, exercise (Nieman, 1999).

The cool down is also an opportunity to introduce relaxation and breathing techniques and all the other elements of programming discussed at the beginning of this section. You can also use the cool down phase to bring the group together socially – stretching, sitting or standing in a circle may encourage people to talk about their plans for the day, what they hope to achieve etc. You can also highlight the other activities at your club or encourage more social activity by organising a coffee together. These small touches will make a difference to how your older adult members interact, and will influence their social connection. A group or class situation is a great opportunity for people to share ideas, get support and advice and get a sense of belonging.

> *Functional training* refers to exercise or activities that reflect the activities of daily living, and is not just focused on fitness gains.

> A programme for older adults should include aerobic endurance, strength, flexibility and balance training.

Aerobic Endurance

The changes in aerobic capacity that are outlined in Part One can severely affect the quality of life for older adults. Simple tasks like getting dressed can be exhausting because of the decline in VO_2 max. Fortunately, aerobic endurance training can make a vast difference and provides the greatest protection against the physiological changes of ageing. Older adults need to begin with low intensity activities and progress to moderate intensity activities to gain maximum benefits. Aerobic endurance training can slow down age related physiological changes, reverse atrophy from disuse, help to control chronic conditions, promote psychological health and preserve the ability to perform activities of daily living (ACSM, 1998).

Training variables for aerobic endurance training

Recommendations for progression

Progression should be slow, ensure a gradual adaptation to the exercise and should not cause any discomfort, pain or injury. The increased risk of chronic disease can have greater consequences for over training, and older adults can take longer to recover.

Older adults can become anxious when intensity or speed is increased and it is recommended that you:

- progress training variables one at a time
- increase time before intensity.

Functional training

When designing an aerobic endurance programme for older adults, consideration must be given to the functional relevance of the exercise programme and how it will benefit their activities of daily living such as shopping, walking up a hill or the stairs. Aerobic endurance can be built up gradually, first by increasing the time and then by increasing the intensity. When working with frail or previously very sedentary participants it may be necessary to start with as little as three minutes a day. For general health, you should aim for at least 30 minutes of moderate intensity physical activity on five or more days a week.

The aerobic exercise mode you select for your client will be guided by the findings of the Physical Activity Readiness Questionnaire (Par Q) that you will have completed (see page 69). Think about your clients' physical condition, lifestyle goals, and their social and psychological needs.

Important considerations

It is very important that you consider the following factors when developing a programme:

- health and training benefits in relation to the client's physical needs for regaining or retaining physical function and reducing the risk of falls in the long term.
- are there any risks involved in the programme, such as aggravating chronic conditions like diabetes or arthritis (see Part Three for more information on chronic conditions).
- consider how the programme will reduce the

Table 4.2	FITT principles and older adults – components of fitness programmes				
	Lifestyle/daily living tasks	Aerobic endurance	Strength	Flexibility	Balance
Frequency/days of week	5–7	5–7	2–3	2–7	3–7
Intensity	Moderate RPE 11–15 (somewhat hard).	RPE 11–15 (40–50 per cent heart rate max).	70–80 per cent of 1RM (be aware this may be quite low in some older adults).	To the point of resistance and gently increase range until mild muscular tension, but no pain, is felt.	Increase difficulty by decreasing base of support using a foam base or stability ball.
Time	The goal is 30 minutes of activity that can be accrued, and can include the various tasks of daily living.	Aim to build up to 30 minutes, but begin with as little as 3–5 minutes if so dictated by you client's fitness, and alternate bursts of activity with active rest. See *interval training* outlined below.	1–3 sets of 10–12 repetitions (the maximum amount of resistance the client can control during one repetition).	10–30 seconds. Progress to a longer time if desired.	5–10 minutes.
Type	Housework, gardening, shopping, walking, washing the car and any activity that uses large muscle groups.	Any activity that uses large muscle groups. Aerobic endurance activities popular with older adults include walking, stationary cycling, treadmill walking or jogging, dancing, swimming, aqua aerobics and exercise to music.	Adapt to strength of client and use own body resistance, seated exercise for extra support, hand weights or dyna bands if more appropriate.	Static yoga stretches.	Tai Chi Yoga poses.

risk of chronic disease, prevent further decline or possibly reverse the spiral of decline (see Part One for more information on physiological changes).
• help your client to plan their rest and recovery time pre- and post-exercise, and build it into the programme you create.
• muscle soreness and fatigue from over-exertion will soon discourage your client. Advise them not to over-exert themselves prior to their session and encourage them to take some time before their session to prepare mentally and physically.
• encourage your client to make time for relaxation post-exercise. In a group you can allow for time at the end of the class to lead a relaxation for 10–15 minutes. For clients in a gym environment, five minutes spent on breathing techniques can be a pleasant way to lift the mood and calm the heart rate (see Part Four for breathing and relaxation techniques).

Table 4.3	Assessing the aerobic endurance training needs of your older clients
Aerobic endurance	• screen for medical conditions and current activity levels in daily and leisure activities. • try to get a measure of the total activity your client does in a day, and average for a week. This will guide your decisions on the intensity and duration on which you base your initial programme. • establish goals that will meet with the functional needs of the client. • review how any chronic conditions will affect the training and consider any adaptations you may have to make (see Part Three) • discuss the social needs of your client. Would they prefer to be in a group, or do they prefer one to one, time out for themselves or a combination? • decide what type of training is most appropriate; gym based, group class, interval training or aqua aerobics.
Special considerations	• monitor how chronic conditions affects exercise response. Older adults may be anxious about increasing intensity and speed for fear of falling. • only progress one exercise variable at a time (increase time or type or intensity). • increase time before intensity.
Measurement and evaluation	• teach your client Borg's RPE scale (see page 34). • encourage your client to record their RPE scales against any activity that they participate in. This will guide you in advising their progression and improve adherence.
Plan, rest and recovery	• always use pre- and post-exercise (see relaxation and breathing techniques on pages 157–60).

Older people can be put off exercising if they over exert themselves and feel uncomfortable, and especially if they suffer an injury.

Interval training

Interval training alternates periods of exercise with equal lengths or longer of *active recovery*. Interval training is ideal for older adults, as it is a flexible framework that can progressively increase endurance training for older adults and is suitable for a broad range of fitness levels. It also reflects real life demands for short bursts of energy during everyday tasks such as hurrying to catch a bus, running out of the rain or walking around a shopping centre. The main advantages of interval training for participants of all ages is that the alternating levels of intensity with active recovery provides a longer and harder workout, but with greater comfort. Another important aspect is that your clients (once they understand Borg's scale on page 34) can control the intensity of the exercise.

Interval allows time for progression and gradually extends periods of aerobic endurance. The recommendations for increases are increments of one minute for as long as your client feels comfortable (Singh, 2000).

Table 4.4	Interval training progressing to continuous training
Please refer to table 11.1 on page 128 for more details on the phases of cardiac rehabilitation.	

Warm up – 15 minutes	
Interval training	*Continuous training*
Alternate periods of maximal effort with short periods of active rest – 2 minutes CV station and 2 minutes active rest. **Time** – depends on fitness level of individual. For example, cardiac rehabilitation phase 3 begins with 1 minute on each, and gradually extends aerobic endurance time by adding 1 minute of walking around the room after each active rest.	Uninterrupted activity performed at a constant sub-maximal intensity. **Time** – build up to 30 minutes continuous CV training at a pace that progresses fitness comfortably for the client.
Active recovery examples – bicep curls, lateral arm raises, upright rows using body bars, side bends, tricep kickbacks, chest press on wall. *N.B. Provide different levels of intensity at each station to suit different levels.*	As active rest decreases, a resistance programme can be introduced after the CV conditioning phase.
Cool down – 10 minutes	
Static stretches working on all muscle groups	
Relaxation	

Table 4.5	Interval training for aerobic endurance for the older adult			
Fitness Level	Number of intervals	RPE and METS* guidelines	Duration	Exercise mode
Deconditioned For older adults just getting started on an activity programme	The number of cycles depends on your client's fitness level, and the length of effort phase	RPE guidelines 9–11 METS guideline 2–4	10 seconds up to 5 minutes for both effort and active recovery phase	Walking, stationary cycling, stair climbing and descending
Moderate to high For clients who are gaining the benefits of regular activity and want to increase their fitness	The number of cycles depends on your client's fitness level, and type of aerobic endurance exercise	RPE guidelines during effort 11–13; progress to 13–15 Active recovery RPE 9–11 METS guideline 4–6; progress to 6–8	Aerobic endurance 3–5 minutes Anaerobic 80–90 seconds; progress to 90–270 seconds Active rest 3–5 minutes	Walking, jogging, cycling, rowing, swimming, exercise to music, circuit training
High For clients who are getting even fitter and want to be fit for sport	The number of cycles depends on your client's fitness level and type of exercise	RPE guidelines during effort 13–15; progress to 15–17 Active recovery RPE 9–11 METS guideline 6–10; progress to 10–12	Aerobic endurance 3–5 minutes Anaerobic 80–90 seconds; progress to 90–270 seconds Active rest 3–5 minutes	Timed or race walks, runs, swims, triathlons, mini marathons

RPE recommendations extracted from *Interval Conditioning Training Continuum for Older Adults* (Brooks, 1995; Dinan and Skelton, 2000) Reference: *Physical Activity Instruction of Older Adults* (Jones and Rose).
*A MET is the Metabolic Equivalent Unit and is a unit to estimate the cost of physical activity. One MET equals oxygen consumption at rest which is approximatly 3.5 millilitres of oxygen per kg of body weight per mintue (3.5ml/kg- 1/min-1).

Interval training vs. interval conditioning vs. continuous training

Interval training alternates periods of exercise of the participant's RPE with equal lengths or longer of active recovery. Interval conditioning provides a flexible framework that can progressively increase aerobic endurance training for older adults, and is suitable for a broad range of fitness levels. It also reflects real life demands for short burst of energy during everyday tasks.

The advantage of interval conditioning for older adults is that the periods of alternating cardiovascular endurance with an active recovery provides an extended and demanding workout, while keeping your client within their comfort zone both psychologically and physically. Interval training is a safe and effective way to improve CV and functional fitness.

After an initial period of interval conditioning (12–16 weeks), as long as there is a progression of aerobic endurance you can encourage your client to extend their training to include continuous training.

Active recovery is training at a low intensity and volume to allow time for recovery from periods of exertion at moderate to high intensity.

Summary

- aerobic endurance training improves VO_2 max and functional ability despite the physiological decline with age, and can make a big difference to quality of life.
- progression should be very gradual, change only one exercise variable at a time and increase duration before intensity.
- rest and recovery time before, during, after and in-between bouts of activity are the keys to minimising the risk of discomfort or injury, and will improve adherence to the exercise programme.
- interval training that alternates periods of exercise with active recovery can provide a safe and progressive exercise format for developing aerobic endurance and progressing to continuous training.
- active recovery training is exercise at low intensity and volume to allow time for recovery from periods of moderate to high intensity exertion.

Resistance training

Research has shown that gains in strength of between 32 and 227 per cent can be achieved after eight or more weeks of resistance training.

Resistance training for older adults can increase muscle hypertrophy and will improve physical function that will significantly enhance their quality of life. It can improve physical function for clients who are living with chronic conditions and diseases such as arthritis, lower back pain, coronary heart disease, stroke and diabetes. It is never too late to begin a resistance training programme and there can be positive gains for even the frailest of older adults. Resistance training is an essential component of an exercise programme for an older adult and will increase the likelihood of retaining independence and autonomy. Many of the physiological changes (see Part One) that occur with age can, in part, be put down to lack of use and a sedentary lifestyle. Resistance training can improve strength, endurance, posture, speed, agility, power and balance for a range of leisure pursuits and activities of daily living.

Table 4.6	Assessing resistance training needs for older adults
Resistance programme composition	• aim to meet the functional training goals of the client • consider how medical conditions and current fitness status affect the programme • include at least one exercise for all the major muscle groups for overall muscular balance • include a combination of single joint (e.g. bicep curl) and multiple joint (e.g. squat) exercises • include a combination of concentric, eccentric and isometric stretches (see the box on page 43) • correct technique is a priority over progression
Exercise sequence – start with large muscle groups and higher intensity exercises, progressing to single joint exercises to reduce fatigue and maximise training quality and duration	• **sets** 1–3 • **reps** 12–15 reps for muscular endurance. For strength a resistance that enables 8–12 reps • **load** 1RM is a safe way to assess older adults • **frequency** short rest periods of 1–2 minutes will enhance muscular endurance 2–3 times a week with a minimum of 48 hours recovery. Beginners may need 2–3 days' recovery time
Special considerations	• older adults may take longer to recover, and progression can be improved by manipulating the different training variables; sets, reps, load and frequency • be aware of any chronic conditions that may affect strength training • have clear aims that meet with the lifestyle goals of the client and any medical conditions • decide if the aim of an exercise is to achieve muscle strength, power or endurance • measurement and evaluation of the resistance programme will provide the instructor with guidance on progression and feedback, reward the client and keep them motivated. Record and monitor body composition and functional ability (i.e. range of movement, sets, load, repetitions achieved and the exercise response on chronic conditions)
Health and safety	• always begin with a warm up of at least 10 minutes • always begin with low resistance • exercise through full **pain free** range of movement • be vigilant with technique and make sure there is no hyperextension or locking of joints

Stretching basics

- a concentric stretch is when the muscles and tendons shorten (e.g. upward phase of bicep curl).
- an eccentric stretch is when the muscles and tendons lengthen (e.g. bicep during lowering phase).
- an isometric stretch is when the muscle remains the same length on the resistance against an immovable object.

When you are developing a strength training programme for a beginner who may be frail or have very weak muscles, the balance of the exercise variables (speed, sets, reps, intensity/load, rest and frequency) needs to be carefully considered to avoid injury or pain. In some cases you may find that fixed weight machines may be too heavy for some older clients, even when on the minimum weight. The weight increments on some resistance machines may be too much for a progression, and other resistance equipment such as free weights bands, body bars, medicine balls, dyna bands and own body resistance may be the starting point to develop a resistance programme. Using a range of resistance equipment and methods will provide both variation in the way you stress the muscles and interest for your client, allowing you to get the best results as you expand and develop their programme.

Training variables for resistance training

The following training variables outline the recommendations to gain a specific training effect. The type of training you select will be guided by the goals of your clients' exercise programmes and their fitness levels.

Loads

- loads that are equal to 90 per cent of 1RM are heavy
- loads that are equal to 70–80 per cent of 1RM are moderate
- loads that are less than 70 per cent of 1RM are light

According to research, even frail elderly adults of 90 years of age are able to tolerate loads of at least 80 per cent of 1RM.

Be aware that heart rate and blood pressure can be elevated by resistance training, especially as the client will experience fatigue at the end of a set of repetitions.
Clients with cardiovascular disease or high blood pressure will need to be monitored.

Functional training

Functional training refers to exercise and activities that reflect the activities of daily living, and is not just focused on fitness gains. Functional training for older adults will stimulate the movement and action of muscles such as twisting, bending, reaching, turning and stepping that are required for daily tasks, for example, stepping up onto a bus or bending down to pick up something off the floor. Examples of specific exercises for functional training can be found in table 4.8 on page 45 and table 4.9 on page 47.

Functional resistance training

Functional resistance training uses a variety of body positions on a range of different surfaces (see balance training on page 52) and uses different resistance equipment such as bands, balls, cable and pulley systems to improve function for daily living activities, for example looking over the shoulder when driving,

Table 4.7	Training variables for resistance training				
Sets	Reps	Intensity/ load	Speed	Rest	Frequency
Proceed with caution for sedentary beginners, with the aim of training for overall body and muscular hypertrophy.					
1–3	8–12	60–80 per cent 1RM	slow to moderate	1–2 minutes between sets	2 x weekly; minimum 48 hours rest
Training for power (for pushing, pulling, leisure activities such as bowling and racket sports)					
1–3	6–10	40–60 per cent 1 RM	high		2–3 x weekly
Muscular endurance					
1–3	10 +	60–80 per cent	moderate	30–60 seconds	2–3 x weekly

picking something up that has dropped on the floor, reaching into cupboards, gardening and housework.

Core stability

Core stability that develops the stability of the trunk muscles, is the foundation for resistance training and will:
- improve ability and technique for functional training
- reduce the risk of injury
- assist performance in all areas of exercise training
- improve ability and stability in daily activities.

Summary

- resistance training can add quality to the life of older adults and increase their enjoyment of a range of leisure, social and daily living activities
- functional training applied to daily living activities will develop stability for balance and mobility for movement
- strength and muscular endurance training will enhance all areas of daily living including work, domestic and leisure and self care
- resistance training will prevent muscle atrophy and aid weight management.

Table 4.8	The benefits of strength training on activities of daily living (ADLs)	
Group muscle	Exercise	ADL benefits
Upper back and Shoulders *Latissimus dorsi, trapezius and deltoids*	• lateral raises • vertical row • dumbbell row • dumbbell flyes • lat pull down	Improves posture and alignment. Improves ability to reach up to shelves in supermarkets and into cupboards, dressing, housework, gardening
Chest *Pectorals*	• chest press • pec dec • dumbbell flyes	Improves strength for lifting, carrying and shopping
Abdominals *Rectus abdominus, obliques*	• abdominal curl • oblique crunch	Core stability, balance and posture control. Supports lower back. Strengthens body for physical activities such as swimming, golf and gardening
Lower back	See Part Three Chapter 7	
Legs *Quadriceps, hamstrings and gluteals*	• leg press • squats • step ups • leg curls • leg extension • lunges	Improved walking technique, balance and moving from sitting to standing
Hip abduction *Inside of thigh*	Can be seated without resistance: • cable pulley • side leg raises; lying or standing; with or without support using dyna bands for added resistance • cable pulley • side steps • double side steps • grapevine	Improved walking technique, balance, agility and stability. Improved balance in movement (dynamic balance). Manoeuvring through crowds with frequent changes of movement e.g. busy supermarket. Other leisure activities such as tennis, badminton
Hip abduction *Outside of thigh*	• side steps • double side steps • grapevine • all of the above in different planes of movement and direction	

Table 4.8	The benefits of strength training on activities of daily living (ADLs) cont.	
Group muscle	Exercise	ADL benefits
Triceps	• tricep kickback • single cable extension using free arm to stabilise working arm • seated dumbbell extension • tricep dips	Lifting and carrying
Biceps	• arm curl • dumbbell curl • seated with dyna bands • cable pulley	Lifting and carrying
Calf raises	• seated or standing	Walking and balance, stability and mobility

Flexibility training

Muscle flexibility and joint mobility training is important for all age groups, and particularly so for older adults, as research has shown that flexibility decreases significantly with age. A loss of flexibility reduces range of movement, increasing the risk of injuries and falls for older adults. Increased stiffness is a part of the ageing process because joint tendons and ligaments which connect muscle to the skeleton become stiffer and less elastic with age. Connective tissue also increases because collagen fibres that make up connective tissue begin to cross link.

This is why range of movement becomes more restricted and will eventually affect stride length, confidence in 'stepping out' in walking and can also lead to a reluctance to be active. See Part One for more on the physiological effects of ageing on flexibility. Flexibility training will improve the lubrication of joints, lower the risk of injury and will help strengthen the tendons and ligaments and maintains the elasticity that will help stabilise the joints. Recommend that your clients do 10–15 minutes of stretching and mobility exercises every day, even when they do not attend a class or training session in the gym.

Muscle Group or Joint	ADL benefits
Table 4.9	**The benefits of flexibility on activities of daily living (ADLs)**
Ankle strengthener (see figures 4.1 & 4.2 on page 48)	Exercises the muscles of the ankle to improve strength for walking and maintaining balance.
Achilles stretch (see figure 4.3 on page 49)	Stretches the Achilles tendon and the lower calf muscle to help maintain flexibility of the ankle for walking, stabilising balance and correct gait.
Hamstring stretch (see fig 4.4 on page 49 for seated option)	Improves and maintains flexibility of hamstrings and glutes needed for walking and general mobility.
Quad stretch (see fig 4.5 on page 50 for seated option)	Improves and maintains flexibility of front of legs required for walking and general mobility and also provides stability for bending and leaning forward.
Lower back stretch	Relieves tension and pain in the back and improves mobility for twisting, turning, bending and reaching.
Hip stretches	Maintains and improves hip mobility for walking and manoeuvring freely through crowded areas, getting in and out of cars or stepping up onto buses.
Oblique stretch (see fig 4.6 on page 50)	Provides a release for muscle on side of trunk and improves mobility for dressing and reaching over head.
Triceps and shoulder stretch	Upper body mobility for dressing, reaching behind and styling hair.
Chest stretch	Improves posture and upper body.
Shoulder stretch	Improves upper body mobility for dressing, reaching behind, reaching.
Triceps stretch	Upper body mobility for dressing, reaching.
Neck stretch	Relieves tension and pain and improves mobility for all tasks of daily living.
Hand flexion (see fig 4.7 on page 51	Strengthens and stretches the fingers through comfortable range of movement to improve and maintain agility and grip for activities such as shopping, cooking, gardening and housework.

Figure 4.1 Standing ankle strengthener

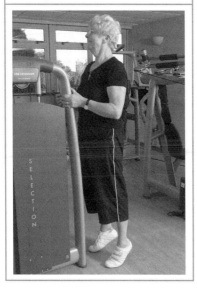

- using wall or bar for support, rise up onto the toes
- hold for 8 counts
- lower heels to floor
- repeat x 4.

Figure 4.2 Seated ankle strengthener

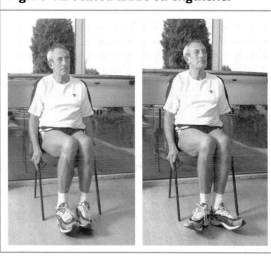

- sit back into chair for support
- sit tall with a long spine and good posture
- thighs are together and knees bent with feet apart
- keep knees together, heels stay on the floor and toes lift up towards the knees – this is the starting position
- rotate both feet inwards, lifting toe towards the knees so toes point towards each other – hold for a few seconds
- place feet on floor and gently slide feet along back to start position
- build up repetitions as ankle strength increases.

Figure 4.3 Achilles stretch

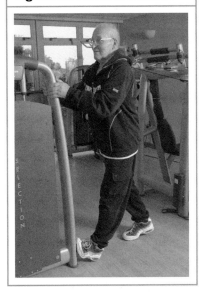

Figure 4.4 Seated hamstring stretch

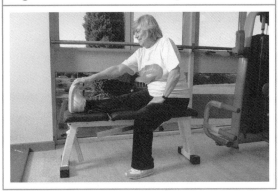

- in a seated position stretch one leg along a bench while the other leg remains on the floor
- keeping a long spine reach forward
- increase the stretch by leaning forward
- hold for 10–15 seconds.

- stand on heels while holding onto a bar or piece of equipment
- lean forward until a mild tension is felt in the back of the leg near the ankle
- stretch can be increased if toes lift higher against a board or piece of equipment and decrease if lowered
- hold for 10–15 seconds.

Figure 4.5 Seated quad stretch

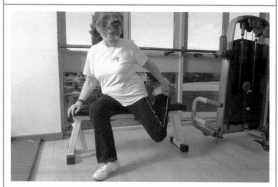

- sit sideways on a chair or bench facing right
- take left leg back until knee points towards the floor until a stretch is felt in the thigh
- lean back to increase the stretch
- hold for 15–30 seconds
- repeat on the left side.

Figure 4.6 Oblique stretch

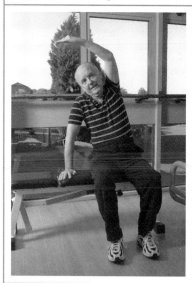

- sit or stand, and lift one arm over the head until a stretch is felt on the side of the body
- you can increase the stretch by resting elbow or forearm on the bench next to the body
- hold for 15–30 seconds.

Figure 4.7 Hand flexion

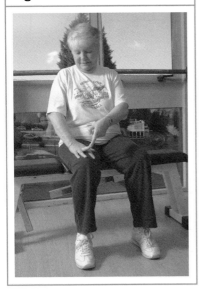

- sit on a bench or chair, place palm of hand on thigh
- using the free hand, gently lift the index finger to its full range of movement and within the comfort zone, holding for 10–15 seconds
- repeat with each finger and thumb
- squeeze hand into a fist and then stretch fingers and hands wide a few times
- finish with a rotation of the wrists right and left.

BALANCE AND MOBILITY TRAINING FOR OLDER ADULTS

5

The ability to balance is a skill that needs to be frequently reviewed, and like any other training it is specific to the task. If you want to take part in a marathon you run, if you want to regain or retain stable balance you have to challenge balance progressively and regularly.

The aim of this section is to provide you with an understanding of why it is important to include an element of balance and mobility training in your exercise programming and classes for older adults. Instructors and personal trainers have an important role to play in the prevention of falls, and you are in a position to reduce the risks of your clients' falling in later life by including balance and mobility training as a specific component of your class structure or exercise programme. The added benefits of doing so are:

- educating your clients and raising awareness that balance and mobility training is a priority for long-term wellbeing and independence
- providing an intervention that can influence the disability and mortality rates that are caused by an injury after a fall
- having a positive impact on a vital area of fitness for older adults.

Teachers of Yoga and Tai Chi will be aware how vulnerable people of all ages are when there is a need to shift and move around while trying to keep balanced. You are likely to find that many of your clients will be surprised at their lack of balance in certain environments and conditions, regardless of age. Most people's ability to balance

goes unchallenged, and it tends to be taken for granted until a fall and injury shocks them into action.

The information on pages 52–3 will tell you more about the physiological changes that affect balance. This section will provide you with information about the different types of balance, how they affect daily activities, specific balance training exercises and their practical application to life. There is also a 'balance exercise guide' (see pages 54–5) for easy reference for you to select, adapt and mould to suit your training programme or class. This is by no means a definitive guide; its purpose is to get you thinking about how the programme you write can improve the quality of life for older adults. If you wish to develop more expertise and broaden your knowledge of falls risk assessment and falls prevention, see the general information section on page 72 for training courses.

What is balance?

Balance is the ability to maintain control on the base of support to avoid falling, and is an essential component of training the over 50s. There are two types of balance; *dynamic balance* and *static balance*.

- **Static balance** is the ability to maintain balance when standing still. Static balance can be improved by challenging the ability to maintain balance and remain still when the base of support is unstable, i.e. standing on a foam base or moving base or sitting on a stability ball. The ability to balance with eyes

Table 5.3	The benefits of balance training on activities of daily living (ADL) cont.	
Balance exercise	Increase the challenge	ADL benefits
Step up and step down	Increase height of step, or use a series of steps with variations in height	Affects climbing up or down stairs and negotiating difficult terrain
Marching on the spot	Knees can be kept low and gradually increase in height	Leg strength and core stability and mobility of the hips for climbing stairs
Striding out	Use different gait lengths and speed – combine with arms and move through different planes of movement	Postural stability and co-ordination, combining tasks of balance with other activities

Ways to incorporate balance training in your programme or class

You should always incorporate 10–15 minutes of balance training into your programme or class, and the list below will give you some ideas about how to approach balance training:

- integrate balance within a circuit as an active rest
- incorporate balance activities in the warm up or cool down
- use stability balls while performing upper and lower body exercises
- in circuits or class situations, give options with varying degrees of difficulty
- increase task demand by performing balance tasks while moving
- encourage pair work in a group exercise session, ball throwing and catching
- create a social atmosphere by working as a group in a circle
- use resistance bands around the hip while partner or instructor increases and releases tension

- design obstacle course that includes objects to step over or move around and include rapid changes of direction
- vary width, length and direction of step
- vary side steps or grapevines from narrow to wider, singles to doubles
- use tape and coloured stickers to mark out straight lines and obstacles
- create imaginary obstacles, for example a river with crocodile-infested waters that your client has to cross by stepping or jumping over the 'crocodiles'. Create a fun atmosphere – older adults are keen to laugh and will appreciate your efforts
- reward effort with praise
- support those who have difficulties and give unconditional respect.

Falls risk assessment

Falls risk assessment is simple to set up and needs minimal equipment. The protocols that follow are typically used to assess senior adults who have a risk of fall and in many cases, after a fall, to assess any future risk. You may want to use the tests to either raise awareness of how important balance training could be in preventing a fall, or perhaps to identify how you could improve balance for an individual client.

1. **Individual assessment** – you should include balance testing as part of the initial screening process for all older adults, especially if you suspect there could be balance difficulties. The results of the test can then inform your decisions on balance or strength training exercises.

2. **In a group setting** – in this setting the aim is for older participants to become more aware of their ability to balance and the importance of working on balance training to reduce risk of falls. The other aim is to create fun around the tests; the purpose is not to compete with others but to have an opportunity to support and socialise with each other.

- the set-up of the tests would be in a circuit
- the group will work in pairs and do the tests together, recording each other's scores
- the scoring is purely to establish a benchmark for themselves and have a reference for repeat tests.

Recording the results

The following score card can be used either by the instructor to record results, or participants to use in a group session.

Table 5.4 Falls assessment score sheet

Name: _____

DOB: _____

Age: _____

Please give details of any medical conditions that may affect your ability and performance in tests, for example arthritis in left knee.

_____

_____

Date	FR inches	CTSIB seconds	30 CS no. of stands	2MMS no. of steps	8ftGO seconds	Chair Sit & Reach	Notes
e.g.	8″	225	15	78	6.4–4.8	2	

Key
FR Functional reach
CTSIB Clinical test for sensory integration and balance
30 CS 30 second chair stand
2MMS 2 minute marching step
8ftGO 8ft up and go

The following protocols can be used for individual testing for balance and aerobic endurance:

Table 5.5	Falls assessment protocols

FUNCTIONAL REACH TEST
(Duncan *et al.*)
The functional reach test provides useful information about dynamic balance control.
Equipment:
- 3 inch x 48 inch yardstick
- small brightly coloured stickers

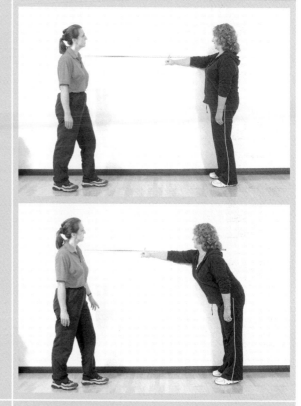

1. Secure a yardstick or tape measure to the wall at shoulder level (specifically at the acromion level) making sure that the measure runs in the direction of the participant's dominant arm.

2. Have a participant stand with feet apart in a comfortable symmetrical position.

3. To make it easier to observe the measurements, attach a bright coloured sticker to the head of the third metacarpal (knuckle of middle finger) on the participant's dominant hand.

4. Get the participant to make a fist (palm down), then raise the reaching arm until it is parallel to the measurement stick. Instruct participant to keep shoulders square by avoiding protracting, retracting or elevating the scapula in this position.

5. The instructor should stand, approximately 4 feet from the participant to record participant's starting position (where the third metacarpal is aligned on the yardstick).

6. Ask participant to reach forwards as far as possible, keeping the fist parallel to the yardstick. Encourage them to use any strategy except touching the surface of the wall or yardstick, holding themselves with the non-reaching hand or taking a step.

Table 5.5	Falls assessment protocols cont.

7. The participant's end reach should be recorded to the nearest ½ inch.

Scoring
- functional reach measurements from 6–10 inches are considered in the normal range
- measurements below 6 inches place the participant in a high risk category for falls related to dynamic balance control
- measurements above 10 inches place the participants in a low risk category for falls related to dynamic balance control.

Common errors in reading functional reach
- failure to observe the 3rd metacarpal of the fisted hand aligned with the yardstick
- evaluator standing at an angle to, rather than directly across from, the yardstick when observing measurement
- participant standing too far from the yardstick of measurement
- poor contrast between the background and measurement markings on the yardstick
- Heels come off the floor when participant leans forward.

NB: *Most individuals should be able to recover a loss of balance during this assessment by stepping forward. However, the recorder should be prepared to assist participants who lose their balance.*

Table 5.5	Falls assessment protocols cont.

THE CLINICAL TEST FOR SENSORY INTEGRATION AND BALANCE (CTSIB)
(A. Shunway-Cook and F.B. Horak)

The CTSIB provides useful information on how well the different sensory systems work together to control balance.

Equipment
• foam
• stopwatch

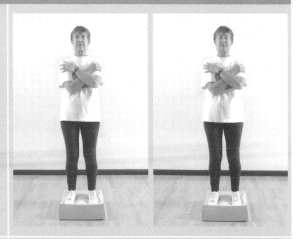

Protocol 1. Firm surface – eyes open

Participant stands on a firm surface (hard floor) with the feet shoulder-width apart, arms crossed over the chest, eyes open, for 30 seconds.

One trial only

Protocol 2. Firm surface – eyes closed

Participant stands on a firm surface (hard floor) with the feet shoulder-width apart, arms crossed over the chest, eyes closed for 30 seconds.

One trial only

Protocol 3. Foam rubber surface – eyes open

Participant stands on 2–4 inch thick foam base with feet shoulder-width apart, arms crossed over chest, eyes open for 30 seconds.

Participant completes trial three times – 30 seconds each.

Scoring
– record the time they were able to hold the position
– if still unable to complete the trial for the full 30 seconds, record the time they were able to hold the

position and do not proceed to the next test level.
– record the time completed for each protocol and note if the trial cannot be completed in proper form.
– completing all four protocols indicates normal balance related sensory system integration.

The total score is the sum of all trials within each protocol.
Score example of an individual able to complete all trials:
Protocol 1 = 30 seconds
Protocol 2 = 30 Seconds
Protocol 3 Trial 1 = 30 seconds, Trial 2 = 30 seconds, Trial 3 = 30 seconds
Protocol 4 Trial 1 = 30 seconds, Trial 2 = 30 seconds, Trial 3 = 30 seconds
Total score 30+30+30 +30+30+30+30+30 = 240

Protocol 4. Foam rubber surface – eyes closed

Participant stands on 2 inch thick foam base with feet shoulder-width apart, arms crossed over chest, eyes closed for 30 seconds.

Participant completes trial three times – 30 seconds each.

Table 5.5   Falls assessment protocols cont.

30 SECOND CHAIR STAND FUNCTIONAL FITNESS TEST

Assesses lower body strength, which is needed to climb stairs, walk distances, get out of a chair, bath or car and rise from sitting or lying down, getting on and off a bus.

Equipment
- stopwatch
- chair (height 17 inches / 43.18 cm, without arms)

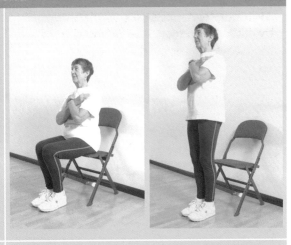

1. Place the chair against a wall or in a secure position so that it does not move during the test.

2. The participant sits in the middle of the chair, feet flat on the floor and arms crossed at the wrist and held against the chest.

3. On the instructor's signal 'GO', the participant rises to a full stand and then returns to a fully seated position.

4. The participant repeats this movement as many times as possible within 30 seconds.

Scoring

Count the number of stands in 30 seconds.

Being more than halfway up at the end of 30 seconds counts as a full stand.

Table 5.5	Falls assessment protocols cont.

AEROBIC ENDURANCE
2 minute marching step functional fitness test

- equipment
- stopwatch
- 30 inch (76cm) piece of cord or string
- 2 inch (5 cm) piece of marking tape
- mechanical counter to help count steps (if possible)

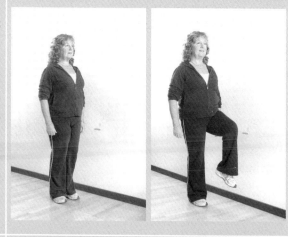

1. On the signal 'GO' the participant begins stepping (not running) in place.

2. Starting with the right leg, the participant completes as may steps as possible within the time period.

3. Both knees must be raised to the correct height to be counted, but the tester counts only the number of times the right knee reaches it.

4. The instructor ensures that the participant maintains proper knee height and also serves as a spotter in case of loss of balance.

5. If proper form cannot be maintained, ask the participant to slow down or rest until proper form can be regained.

6. Keep the stopwatch running; stepping and counting can be continued if the 2 minute period has not elapsed.

Scoring

— measure the height to which you will ask the participant to raise his or her knees.
— find the correct height by stretching a piece of cord from the participant's knee to the top of the hipbone.
— fold the cord in half and mark this spot on the thigh with the tape. Move the participant to a wall and transfer the tape from the thigh to a spot at the same level on the wall. This will allow you to monitor knee height while stepping.

Table 5.5	Falls assessment protocols cont.

THE 8 FOOT UP AND GO FUNCTIONAL FITNESS TEST

(Rikli, Ph.D. and Jessie Jones, Ph.D)

Assesses motor mobility and dynamic balance – important for recovering from tripping, manoeuvring in a crowd and a variety of recreational and sport activities.

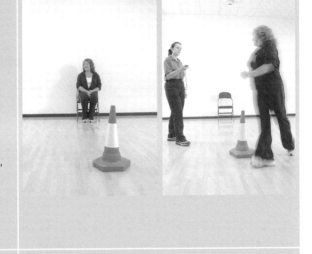

Equipment

- stopwatch
- straight back chair (height 17 inches / 43.18 cm, without arms)
- tape measure
- cone

- Place the chair against the wall or in a secure position so that it does not move during testing.
- Place a cone marker 8ft (2.44 metres) away measured from back of cone to a point on the floor level with the front edge of the chair. There should be at least 4 feet (1.22m) of clearance beyond the cone to allow ample turning room for the participant

Protocol

1. Allow one practice and then complete two test trials

2. The participant sits in the middle of the chair (not on edge) in upright posture

3. Hands on thighs and feet flat on floor

4. One foot can be slightly in front of the other

5. On your signal 'GO' the participant gets up from the chair (pushing of thighs or chair is allowed) and walks (not runs) as quickly as possible around the cone then walks back to the chair and sits down.

Scoring

The instructor starts the timer on 'GO' whether or not the participant has started to move, and stops the timer at the exact moment the participant sits fully in the chair.

Record the best score (fastest time) to the nearest one-tenth of a second.

Table 5.5	Falls assessment protocols cont.

CHAIR SIT AND REACH

Assesses lower body flexibility – important for good posture and normal gait pattern.

Equipment
• chair

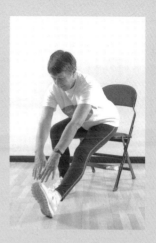

1. The participant takes up a seated position on the front of the chair with leg extended.
2. Reach with hands towards toes

Score

1. reach to middle of extended leg
2. able to reach just past knee of the extended leg
3. able to reach to knee of extended leg
4. able to reach to mid thigh of the extended leg
5. able to reach knee but unable to complete correct technique
6. unable to reach forwards because of pain, deformity or fear of falling.

1–4 no limitation
5   severe limitation
6   unable

Table 5.6	Performance norms						
Age group	60–64	65–69	70–74	75–79	80–84	85–89	90–94
30 SECOND CHAIR STAND (number of stands)							
Women	12–17	11–18	10–15	10–15	9–14	8–13	4–11
Men	14–19	12–18	12–17	11–17	10–15	8–14	7–12
8 FOOT UP & GO (number of seconds)							
Women	6.0–4.4	6.4–4.8	7.1–4.9	7.4–5.2	8.7–5.7	9.6–6.2	11.5–7.3
Men	5.8–3.8	5.7–4.3	8.0–4.2	7.2–4.6	7.6–5.2	8.9–5.3	10.1–6.2
TWO MINUTE MARCHING STEP (number of steps)							
Women	75–107	73–107	68–101	68–100	60–91	55–85	44–72
Men	87–115	86–116	80–110	73–109	71–103	59–91	52–88

Tai Chi, Yoga, Pilates, ball games, throwing, batting, catching, stability ball, chair exercises are all excellent and fun ways to challenge balance and co-ordination

Pilates

Pilates contains gentle exercises without high impact or muscular stress and is frequently recommended to those needing rehabilitation though physical therapy. It is considered a good workout for older adults as it promotes good posture through core stability.

Pilates will strengthen the back and spine, increase mobility of joints and improve circulation. It achieves core conditioning and peripheral mobility through actions that focus on the abdominal muscles, pelvic floor, lower back and scapula regions and can help to improve balance, agility and stability of older adults. Other benefits include improved flexibility, co-ordination and body awareness as well as increased circulation, reduced blood pressure, better joint mobility and improved posture.

Tai Chi

The purpose of Tai Chi is to achieve balance throughout the body with the use of flowing movements and synchronised breathing, bringing the mind and body into harmony. Tai Chi can improve concentration, improve ankle, hip and knee stability and is particularly effective for improving the balance, mobility and co-ordination of older adults.

The art of Tai Chi rests on five basic principles:

1. **relaxation** – applying just enough strength for every movement or task conserves energy and maintains stamina
2. **separating Yin and Yang** – this principle refers to the philosophy of opposites in nature, for example force versus relaxation, speed versus stillness and weight shifts etc.
3. **turning at the waist** – a strong and flexible waist is essential in connecting the upper and lower body
4. **keeping the back erect** – keeping the

body perpendicular to the ground in order to achieve balance, comfort, relaxation and optimal energy

5. **total body involvement** – the ability of the whole body to move together, not limb by limb, comes from applying the first four principles.

> Tai Chi can improve balance, reduce falls and increase leg strength. It also lowers stress hormones, enhances respiratory and immune function and promotes emotional wellbeing. To research more about the benefits of Tai Chi for older adults see the information section on page 67.

Yoga

Yoga is a physical and spiritual discipline that combines specific postures and breathing techniques to enable deep meditation, relaxation and strength. According to yoga philosophy, it is the flexibility of the spine, not the number of years, which determines a person's age. It is said that yoga can slow down the ageing process by enhancing flexibility of the spine, firming the skin, improving muscle tone and correcting posture. The functional benefits are improved flexibility and mobility and will enhance balance and co-ordination.

A combination of yoga breathing, meditation and relaxation can also help to relieve pain. Lower back pain is a common problem that responds well to the strength and flexibility that yoga practice can provide. Practising yoga can also provide chronic pain sufferers with useful tools to actively cope with their pain.

Yoga practice consists of:

- **asanas** (postures) – practising of specific postures provides gentle stretching and movements that increase flexibility and also help to correct bad posture.
- **pranayama** (breathing exercises) – breathing patterns can affect the spine in various ways such as movement of the ribs, and changes pressure within the chest and abdomen. Exhaling can also be used to relax muscles.
- **relaxation and meditation** – relaxation can be an antidote to stress. Visualisation techniques can be used, for example get your clients to imagine a movement before performing it as this can make it easier to move the muscles that are about to be used.

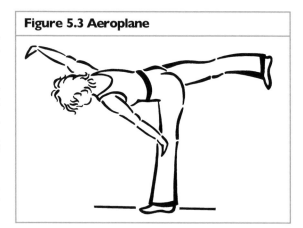

Figure 5.3 Aeroplane

Figure 5.4 Eagle

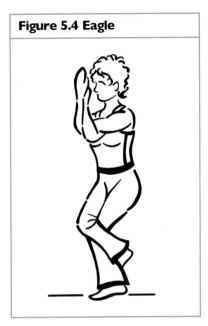

Figure 5.5 Star pose

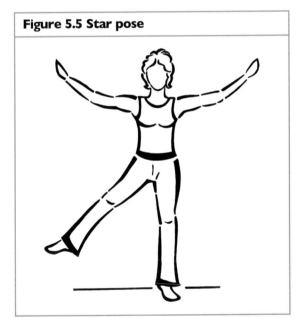

Pre-exercise screening

The Physical Activity Readiness Questionnaire (PAR Q recommended by Skills Active is the Canadian model, which can be viewed on www.csep.ca/forms.asp) is completed by the client and identifies any symptoms of heart disease and musculoskeletal problems that need consideration before taking part in any exercise. It is a very simple questionnaire, will highlight information you need immediately, and it is recommended that you include these questions when you screen clients.

The exercise programme needs will vary considerably with older adults. There are the physiological changes that occur with age (see Part One) and there may be additional complications with chronic conditions (see Part Three). The purpose of screening is to assess a client's individual needs and interests (see Part Four), and gain information about their medical history and any medication that may influence their response to exercise.

The following screening tools will help you assess your client for any contraindications to exercise (conditions where exercise is not recommended). If you find your client is contraindicated, they *must* seek their GP's advice before participating in a class or exercise programme.

Table 5.7	Conditions and symptoms to be considered when screening for contra indications
Refer to a GP for advice and recommendations for exercise if any of the following conditions apply:	
Cardiovascular disease	
Symptoms of cardiovascular disease	
Risk of cardiovascular disease	
A chronic condition that is aggravated by activity or exercise	
Unstable diabetes	
Unstable angina (chest pain)	
Irregular heart beat	
Severely high blood pressure (200/110 or above)	
Symptoms	
Pain or tightness in the chest could be related to heart disease (see Part Three)	
Shortness of breath while at rest or after light activity could indicate obstructed blood flow of the lungs, chronic obstructive pulmonary disease (COPD) or heart disease (see Part Three)	
Fatigue after mild exertion may be a sign of poor blood flow or low oxygen levels in the blood	
Swelling of the ankles may be linked to the heart pumping less blood	
Pain in legs could indicate peripheral artery disease if brought on by exercise	
Dizziness and fainting is a sign of insufficient blood flow to the brain	

Screening tools

The following screening tools will provide you with additional information on your client's health status. They will give you a baseline to measure progress and the effectiveness of your exercise programme, and also be a motivator for clients.

Table 5.8	Screening tools		
Screening tool	*Formula*	*What they measure*	*Reading the result*
Body Mass Index (BMI)	Weight in KGs, divided by height in metres squared. **BMI = KG/m2**	BMI provides information about body weight in relation to height, and can be used to assess if clients are within a healthy range.	Healthy range = 18.5–24.9 Overweight = 25–29.9 Obese = 30 + (and increased risk of heart disease, hypertension and diabetes).
Waist to hip ratio (WHR)	Measure the clients waist circumference at the narrowest point (around the navel) and divide by the measurement of the widest point of the hips. **WHR = waist circumference/hip circumference**	Assesses abdominal fat. High scores indicate an increase in the risk of heart disease, type II diabetes and hypertension.	Measurements above 1.03 for men and 0.90 for women aged 60–69 indicate an increased risk of heart disease. Men with a waist circumference higher than 102 cm (40 ") and women higher than 88 cm (35") **and** have a BMI of 30+ are very high risk for coronary artery disease
Blood pressure	Blood pressure measures systolic pressure (the pressure while the heart contracts) and diastolic pressure (the pressure while the hear relaxes). **BP = Systolic/ Diastolic**	Assess health risk for exercise.	Mild hypertension is diagnosed if systolic pressure is 140 mmHg or higher, and diastolic pressure is 90mmHg or higher. (see Part Three on hypertension on page 129).

Summary

- exercise programmes for older adults need to be planned with the principles of fitness in mind: **specificity, overload, functional relevance, and accommodation**.
- applying the training variables of **frequency, intensity, time and type** in a way that progresses clients comfortably and safely towards their goals will improve adherence to their programme.
- a balanced programme for older adults should include all training components: **aerobic endurance, resistance training, flexibility, mobility and balance training**.
- balance testing to assess falls can help inform your decisions on the type of balance or strength training exercises that are required to improve or maintain balance of older clients.
- balance testing and training older participants to become more aware of their ability to work on balance ability may reduce risk of falls.
- the main objective of pre-exercise screening it to assess the level of risk against the risk factors of older adults, and identify any contraindications for exercise.
- men over 45 and women over 55 who have two or more risk factors need to seek their GP's advice before beginning an exercise programme.
- screening of older adults should be a regular part of the review process. Older adults are at greater risk of developing chronic diseases and periodic screening is recommended, particularly if there are any signs or symptoms as outlined in table 5.7 on page 70.

> 'Old age ain't no place for sissies'
>
> Bette Davis

References

Cress, M. E., Buchner, D. M., Prohaska, T., Rimmer, J., Brown, M., Macera, C., DiPietro, L., Chodzko-Zajko, W. (2004), 'Physical activity programs and behavior counseling in older adult populations', *Medicine and Science in Sports and Exercise*, 3611, 1997–2003.

Jessie Jones, C. and Rose, Debra J. (2005), *Physical Activity Instruction of Older Adults* (Human Kinetics)

Leicester College (2000), *Exercise for Improving Postural Stability and Reducing the Risk of Falls.*

Tortora, G. J. and Grabowski, S. R. (1993) *Principles of Anatomy and Physiology*, seventh edition (Harper Collins)

Online resources

www.laterlifetraining.co.uk, provides specialist, safe and effective exercise training for people working with vulnerable older populations.

TRAINING OLDER ADULTS WITH CHRONIC CONDITIONS

PART THREE

CHRONIC CONDITION EXERCISE GUIDES

6

The aim of this section is to give you the information you need to be able to create a safe and effective exercise programme for older adults living with arthritis, osteoporosis, lower back pain, stroke, chronic obstructive pulmonary disease, diabetes and hypertension. There are guides for each condition that you can use as an easy reference tool to support the advice you give to your client, and they will also assist you in making decisions on the frequency, intensity, time and type of exercises you recommend.

Each part has been designed to make it easy for you to get the information you need quickly and has the following structure:

What is it?

Describes the condition, providing useful information for you to refer to when you are presented with a client that has the condition.

Exercise recommendations

Sets out the fitness goals for that condition, although you are encouraged to explore the goals of the clients and provide a more complete client-centred approach that meets with their needs and also taps into your own creativity.

The components of fitness are clearly separated again for easy access and you will be able to retrieve information for recommendations for cardiovascular training, strength training, flexibility and mobility. At the end of each section you will also find an 'at a glance' summary of exercise recommendations that you can photocopy for easy reference and use when designing your programme. This will be particularly useful when you are working with a client with more than one condition, and you need all the information in front of you.

Special considerations and screening guidelines

Highlights the symptoms and complications of a condition that you need to consider both when you are designing the programme and whenever your client is exercising. The symptoms of chronic conditions can change daily and you will need to be alert to how and when you should adapt a programme, or perhaps recommend that your client should rest or seek medical attention.

Client care and education

Information that you can pass onto your client for their general knowledge, comfort and safety.

Adaptations and modifications

Aims to help you think about how you can monitor and adapt the exercise recommendations to the specific requirements of your client's needs and condition. In an ideal world I would give you a package of 'off the shelf' exercise programmes and in the past I have tried to create them.

However, this is not practical – there are so many exercise variables when working with older adults who may have two or more chronic conditions and a base fitness level ranging from very sedentary beginners to master athletes.

The format of *adaptations and modifications* is different for each condition and provides guidance that is relevant to that condition. Applying the guidance in order to adapt and modify the exercise will require thought, imagination, clear instruction, knowledge and responsibility, and it will be client centred. You may come across a conflict in exercise recommendations when you are writing an exercise programme for a client with two or more chronic conditions. If you have any concerns, seek advice from specialists and medical professionals that can help.

Training older adults with chronic conditions

A chronic condition refers to a disease of long duration that starts slowly and involves slow changes; it does not indicate anything about the severity of a condition, which will vary among clients. The symptoms of a chronic condition can often be relieved by regular activity, providing both the physical and psychological support to help people cope with their condition and improve their quality of life.

Exercise programming for older adults

It is very easy to become very focused on writing a programme *for* the chronic condition, and forget the person who is living with it. This can lead to a client feeling they are a condition that needs to be treated, rather than the individual who is having to deal with it.

When designing an exercise programme for the older adult with a chronic condition, the primary aim of the instructor is to ensure the safety, comfort and enjoyment of the client, while also considering the following health and fitness goals:

- to work towards what the client wants to achieve and what they consider important to their happiness and wellbeing
- to reduce the risk of decline caused by inactivity
- to ease symptoms of chronic condition where possible
- to improve cardiovascular fitness, muscular strength, flexibility and mobility
- to reduce the risk of falls.

Be aware that you may have to manage your client's expectations and guide them towards positive goals and realistic timescales.

To help an older adult with a chronic condition it is really important to think carefully about how the client will experience the programme you design, and take some time to consider the physical and psychological effects of living with a chronic condition. The primary consideration should be that the programme is interesting for the client and is based on what they ultimately want to achieve. The aim is to harmonise the medical goals of the GP, the physical fitness goals of the instructor and the lifestyle goals of the client. It can be useful to explain the health benefits of an exercise programme but if the client just wants to be able to walk to the supermarket and carry their own shopping, then that should be the frame of reference you use when teaching your client their programme. Every programme you design must be a totally personal experience and connect with their motivation to exercise.

A responsible instructor must be very concerned about creating a safe programme that does not aggravate the condition, but this can lead to a client feeling that the focus is on the condition rather than them. It is also important to keep in mind that the person who has the condition is like any 'normal' client – they will want to make the best of themselves and look and feel good too.

Acceptance of the effects of ageing does not come naturally, and personal desires and self image does not automatically adjust when signs of ageing appear, such as when wrinkles and chronic conditions become a part of daily living. As ageing people we do have to make psychological and physical adjustments but that does not mean that we no longer have a desire to feel beautiful, sexy and strong. The skill of the instructor is designing a programme that manages the physical condition while allowing your client to feel capable and motivated towards achieving ***their goals***. Most importantly, you need to help your client ignite that inner glow that reflects back at the world when someone feels good about him or herself.

Working with an older adult who has one or more chronic conditions or physical limitations will require a much more personal approach. You will need to work with the client to adapt and modify exercises due to the limitations caused by a specific condition, while still providing a balanced programme that meets the needs of the client. It is difficult to provide examples of the 'ideal' programme for, say, arthritis, as other conditions or the client's interest may influence you to make other choices. What this section sets out to do is to help you consider how a condition may affect the client's comfort on certain equipment, the mechanics of movement during specific exercises and how they may affect the client physically as well as psychologically.

Five things to consider when writing an exercise programme for a client with a chronic condition:

1. what happens mechanically during an exercise and how will that impact on the condition of your client? You can use diagrams and charts of skeleton and muscles and use visualisation to see how movement affects joint and muscle action.
2. think about the positions of the joints and muscles in relation to the chronic condition, how do the joints and muscles move and how will that affect a chronic condition such as an arthritic hip or chest muscles after heart surgery. Consider how the plane of movement and the position of the body on certain exercise machines may compress or reduce ROM and aggravate the pain of arthritis or osteoporosis.
3. how will it feel to the client – the aim is to make the client confident and at ease. Awkward positions in front of a mirror can make some people feel self-conscious and demotivate them very quickly. Work out with the client and ask yourself what would work best to achieve the health goal of the client, minimise pain and prevent further deterioration.
4. how can you adapt the programme during 'flare ups' and what alternatives or modifications can you suggest? Living with a chronic condition can be debilitating and mentally very wearying, the right kind of programming can help the client feel more in control and psychologically able to cope.
5. The challenge of the fitness instructor is to find solutions to what can be a complex situation with clients that have one or more contraindications that conflict with the exercise required.

Physical activity and chronic pain

Working with older adults increases the likelihood of you working with clients that have a chronic condition, and who may also suffer from chronic pain. Your empathy and understanding will help your client to feel supported and confident. If chronic pain is unmanaged it can become a severe affliction for the sufferer, and can lead to a vicious cycle where the sufferer is so preoccupied with the pain that it results in what is refereed to as the 'terrible triad'; suffering, sleeplessness and sadness.

What is chronic pain?

Chronic pain is a persistent pain that can continue for weeks, months and, in severe cases, even years. The trigger of the pain may have been an accident or injury such as a sprain, or there may be an ongoing cause such as arthritis. Some people can suffer chronic pain for an unidentified reason. Types of treatment for the management of pain include:

- exercise
- stretching
- manipulation and massage
- electrical therapy
- hydrotherapy
- movement and posture training
- advice on managing everyday activities, including work.

Sometimes pain does not go away despite all kinds of therapies and treatments. Continuous pain can affect mood, mobility, self confidence and sleep patterns, which can have an impact on working life, home life and personal and social relationships.

People with chronic pain can be helped by a sympathetic and caring instructor who can provide psychological support and motivation for the client who may be afraid of activity because of the pain. The aim of the instructor in this instance would be to design a suitable programme that will work with the pain, or around it, to prevent muscle atrophy from inactivity.

Chronic conditions

Most older adults, especially those over 65, will have one or more chronic conditions and some functional limitation that will affect their ability to carry out basic activities, for example walking, climbing stairs, shopping, bending, reaching, carrying and lifting. It is important to consider the practical implications of how your exercise programme can improve your client's experience of everyday living, and help them to maintain their physical functioning. Verbrugge & Jette (1994) developed a *disablement process model* that describes how a chronic condition can lead to impairments in other body systems such as cardiovascular, musculoskeletal, cognitive, sensory and motor. For example, a person who has arthritis in the knee is likely to have poor posture, walk less often and more slowly, which can lead to muscle atrophy (musculoskeletal system) and a reduction in their aerobic fitness (cardiovascular system). Over a period of time this can lead to a disability. However, early intervention and an exercise programme designed specifically to address the condition can delay or prevent decline. The research has also found that exercise may even reverse functional decline (Camaione and Owen, 2001).

The spiral of decline

A suitable activity programme can help a person develop the physical and mental strength to cope better with a chronic condition.

Health or physical problem

The spiral of decline can begin with an injury, a disease or chronic condition that affects ability to be freely active because of a limitation that is imposed on an individual. A few examples are the pain of an arthritic joint, the breathlessness of asthma or the recovery from an operation of some kind. Any physical limitation can discourage a person from being active, and lead to a lack of motivation and consequently a deterioration of health and fitness.

Physical limitation leading to inactivity

Enforced or self-imposed inactivity can result from a fear of pain, or of making the condition worse, and can lead to lack of use or over-compensation from other body parts, putting a strain on other systems. Pain in a joint or muscle can lead to bad posture alignment which can then trigger other conditions, such as back problems. Furthermore, when the motivation to be active declines, cardiovascular fitness will deteriorate, muscles atrophy and body weight increase, all of which contribute to a negative mental attitude that can lead to depression.

Discouraged to disability

A depressed person is a demotivated person, and the longer the person remains inactive there is an increased risk of becoming disabled in some way. Tasks of daily living become difficult, and this can result in increased or total absenteeism from work, and social interests and family life being neglected. The focus of the person at the outset of any condition or disease needs to be turned to how an exercise programme can help them mange their health problem and build up the strength and reserve in other body systems to prevent a spiral of decline into disability and depression. However, at any stage a suitable activity programme can help a person develop the physical and mental strength to live with their condition.

Repetitive strain injury

Repetitive strain injury (RSI) is the name often assigned to a group of conditions that are caused when too much strain is placed on a joint, and occurs when the same action is performed over and over. RSI is more common in those over the age of 30, and needs to be

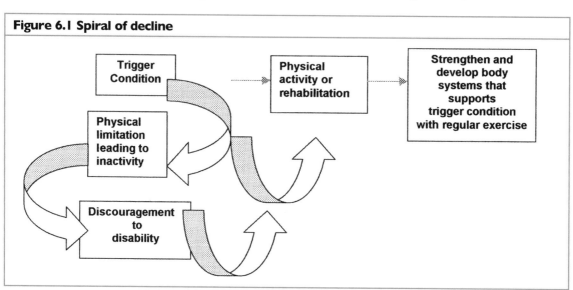

Figure 6.1 Spiral of decline

considered when creating a programme for older adults. Some forms of RSI can be caused or aggravated by chronic conditions or disease such as rheumatoid arthritis, osteoarthritis, and diabetes. Older adults are more susceptible, particularly if they have, or have had, manual jobs. The two most common types of RSI are:

1. **tendinitis** – inflammation of a tendon
2. **bursitis** – inflammation of a bursa (small fluid filled sacs that act as a cushion between tendons and bones).

The symptoms of RSI are:

- pain in one specific area
- a tender, swollen, red or hot area
- a tingling and numbness, coldness or loss of sensation
- a loss of grip strength, lack of endurance, weakness or fatigue
- pain or numbness while lying in bed.

Types of RSI

- **bicipital tendinitis** is inflammation of the tendon that attaches the biceps to the shoulder and is caused by using the arm to make repeated movements such as scrubbing the floor or painting and decorating
- **tennis elbow** is inflammation of the outer border of the elbow caused by over use of the forearm muscles, for example by bending the wrist backwards with force when playing tennis or painting with a brush
- **golfer's elbow** is inflammation of the inside of the elbow caused by repetition of bending the wrist forward with force, for example through golfing or pulling ropes.
- **trigger finger** is inflammation of the tendons in the hands that are used to make a fist and may cause bumps to form on the tendon and the fingers to lock. This will affect ability to grip.

- **DeQuervain's tendosynovitis** is inflammation of the lining that surrounds the tendons in the thumb and is caused by repeated twisting of the wrists.
- **trochanteric bursititis** is inflammation of the bursa on the outer hip.
- **housemaid's knee** is an inflammation of the bursa on the front of the kneecap caused by frequent kneeling for long periods of time, for example during domestic chores and some manual jobs.
- **carpal tunnel syndrome (CTS)** is the compression of the median nerve which runs down the arms to the fingers and causes severe pain that can extend to the neck. CTS is caused by short repetitive movements such as typing and using vibrating tools for long periods of time.

The implications of RSI on exercise for older adults

- older adults are more susceptible to RSI so it is important that the correct technique and form are observed
- it is important that repetitions, or any exercise that involves grip or repetitive joint movement and impact, are gradually increased in number
- variations on type of exercise can also reduce the risk of RSI.

Treatments for RSI

The treatments for people suffering from RSI may include the following:

- non-steroid anti-inflammatory drugs
- moderate exercise to help strengthen the joint (although only if there is no pain and swelling, and excessive repetition is avoided)
- relaxation of the muscles around the inflamed area (see pages 157–60 for breathing and relaxation techniques).

Brenda's case study

I was thirty-eight and going through a very painful divorce when a friend nagged me to take some squash lessons. I booked them with the local sports centre and went along only to be told that I needed to build myself up, get strong and put some weight on. I decided to take circuit training classes and it wasn't long before I was attending three circuits and two aerobic classes a week. I felt great – full of confidence and alive.

The exercise changed over the years and when I got to fifty my knees became very painful, I was gaining weight fast and mentally feeling old with aching joints and tight clothes. I had my knees x-rayed and the pain turned out to be deferred pain from two worn vertebrae in my lower back. My fears were that I would become like my mum who is very overweight and crippled with arthritis. I had a very demanding desk job so I would be sitting down all day and would often stay late. When I did get home I would eat late and go to bed. What had happened to my exercise routine? It had gone, and I felt that I was on a hamster wheel and my back pain was getting worse. I had some physiotherapy, and quickly realised that I had to look very carefully at my eating habits and start an exercise programme.

For the last eight years I have kept to a regular exercise routine. I take spinning classes three times a week before work as this helps me burn calories and improve my cardiovascular fitness, without the pressure on my joints. I do two 'Body Pump' classes a week to improve my bone density and keep me toned, and I also attend 'Body Balance' classes twice a week for my strength and flexibility.

Combined with healthy eating, this plan works very well for me. I have made sure that my exercise routine works well with my life – either on the way to work or on the way home, five days a week. If I have a day off I don't feel guilty because I know that I'll be there tomorrow. Now at 55 I am able to manage my back problems, I feel great, and I think that I look good too!

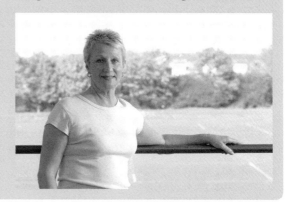

CHRONIC CONDITIONS OF THE MUSCULOSKELETAL SYSTEM

7

The majority of older adults over the age of 65 will be experiencing some kind of joint ache and pain, and the most common causes will be arthritis and lower back pain. Arthritis is a degenerative joint disease caused by wear and tear, or an auto immune disease caused by the immune system attacking healthy tissue and damaging joints. It is very important for older adults who have arthritis to be active and mobile, as a sedentary lifestyle will make their condition worse and they could spiral into a decline of disability and dependence (see the *spiral of decline* figure on page 78). Lower back pain affects all age groups and can become chronic for older people who have arthritis of the spine.

Arthritis can be a very painful condition, and will vary between individuals – with some clients experiencing mild discomfort and others experiencing severe discomfort, leaving them limited in their range of movement. The extent to which a client can take part in any kind of activity will depend on their pain threshold. People with higher pain thresholds will be able to do more, although it is important that the programme always remains *within* the client's pain threshold.

Arthritis

What is arthritis?

Arthritis is a rheumatic disease that causes pain, stiffness and swelling that affects joints and limits the range of movement of the joint. The two most common types of arthritis are:

1. **Osteoarthritis (OA)** is a degenerative joint disease resulting in a gradual loss of joint cartilage affecting one or two joints, mostly weight-bearing joints such as hips, spine, knees, and fingers and toes.
2. **Rheumatoid arthritis (RA)** is inflammation of the synovial fluid that lines the joints causing swelling. RA is an auto immune disease in which the body attacks its own tissues such as cartilage and joint linings, causing inflammation of the joint, swelling, pain and loss of function. Clients with rheumatoid arthritis need to rest from exercise during painful flare-ups.

Exercise is important for clients with arthritis to help them maintain a reasonable range of movement, and reduce the health risk associated with inactivity. Improved aerobic capacity, endurance, strength, and flexibility are associated with improved function, decreased joint swelling and pain. Increased social and physical activity in daily life can reduce depression and anxiety.

Exercise recommendations

Goals

To improve or maintain cardiovascular fitness and muscular strength, and provide stability for affected joints. To maintain or improve range of movement to reduce stiffness. To improve core stability and balance.

Cardiovascular (CV) training

The exercise programme needs to be low to moderate intensity with gradual progression. If necessary for the comfort of the client, take an accumulative approach and break the session down into activities that can be carried out throughout the day. Put the goal emphasis on time and building up the duration, rather than distance or intensity. For example, 3 x 10 minute sessions working towards 2 x 15 minute sessions. Use low impact aerobics non-weight-bearing exercises to avoid excessive joint stress, for example swimming, water aerobics, chair exercise and cycling. Treadmill walking is also an option if the client is comfortable, and the impact is not too hard on the arthritic knees, hips and toes. Try with a gradient of 1–2 per cent, which softens the footfall slightly and will reduce the impact (however, do watch your client's posture as they may compensate by leaning forwards). Gradually build the duration from as little as 3 minutes (as the client's ability dictates) to 30 minutes with interval training (see pages 38–40 for interval conditioning guidelines). Aim to progress frequency to 5 sessions per week, and include activities outside of the gym or studio environment such as walking, gardening and domestic chores.

Strength training

Strength training needs to be included to increase muscle strength to support and protect arthritic joints. Dyna bands, free weights and resistance machines are all suitable. Your selection will depend on which joints are affected, how it affects your client's grip as well as how weight-bearing the exercise is on the arthritic joint. If any exercise is too painful then replace them with isometric or static strength exercises (where a muscle develops tension without changing length or angle of the joint). Straight leg exercises are a good way to strengthen the leg muscles around an arthritic knee, although avoid locking out at the knee. Include posture training to improve slouched positions that may compress joints and aggravate the condition (see pages 77–80 for guidance on chronic pain)

> Be aware that isometric contractions produce significantly higher systolic and diastolic blood pressures and may not be advisable for clients with hypertension, coronary heart disease, or stroke.

Flexibility and range of movement (ROM)

Stretching and joint mobilisation should be done daily (including flare-up days, although avoid other exercise until the flare-up has subsided). Start with a small range of movement and gently increase the stretches until mild muscular tension is felt. Resistance machines on the lightest weights can also be used for controlling the range of movement in some mobility exercises and provide a support for your client.

Special considerations and screening guidelines

- joint range of movement may be restricted by stiffness, swelling, and pain and may affect the client's ability with regard to walking speed and cycle revolutions.
- make sure that correct technique is followed and that all movements are controlled, as there is a high risk of injury from de-conditioned muscles and poorly supported joints.
- highly repetitive movements should be avoided for extended periods., for eaxample group cycle or rowing classes.
- avoid morning exercise for clients with rheumatoid arthritis due to morning stiffness,

and complete rest is advisable during painful flare-ups.
- if pain or swelling appears or persists, reduce load on joint, or stop exercise completely.

Client care and education

✓ warm up before exercise, and if desired, apply ice packs after exercise
✓ avoid jarring ballistic movements
✓ plan for exercise by not over-exerting yourself prior to class or training
✓ work according to your level of ability
✓ modify your exercise during an arthritic flare up
✓ rest if the joint inflammation is acute red, hot swollen, painful
✓ buy trainers with good shock absorption to protect joints
✓ stretch daily including flare-up days, but avoid other exercise until the flare-up has subsided.

Adaptations and modifications (cardiovascular training)

> Bear in mind at all times when working with clients who have arthritis, there will almost always be some level of pain to tolerate, so be patient and supportive.

When you are preparing a cardiovascular programme for a client who has arthritis you will need to know what type of arthritis they have, and the joints that are affected. Most commonly affected are weight-bearing joints – hips, spine, knees, fingers and toes. Your first consideration when selecting the equipment and specific exercises is what happens to the affected joint when it carries out the movement of the exercise. Does the angle of the movement at the joint reduce space around the joint or does the movement allow for space around the joint so it can move relatively freely?

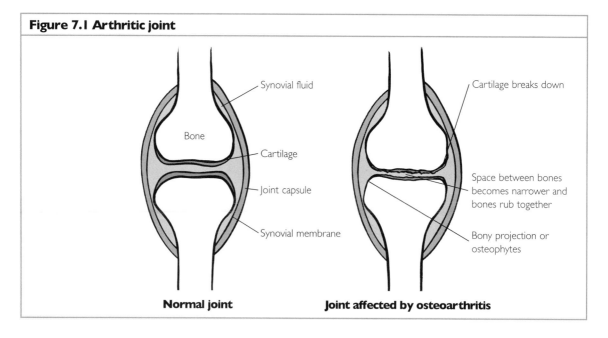

Figure 7.1 Arthritic joint

Synovial fluid

Bone

Cartilage

Joint capsule

Synovial membrane

Cartilage breaks down

Space between bones becomes narrower and bones rub together

Bony projection or osteophytes

Normal joint

Joint affected by osteoarthritis

Upright bike

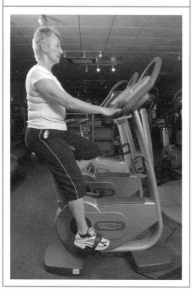

Figure 7.2 Correct position on upright bike

- correct upper body posture helps to prevent pressure bearing down, and lifts the torso up and away from the hip joint
- the weight bears down on the glutes, and the action of cycling pushes down away from the hip and opens up the joint
- for clients with arthritis in the knee you can take the saddle seat higher, reducing the bend at the knee and opening up the angle of the joint.

Recumbent bike

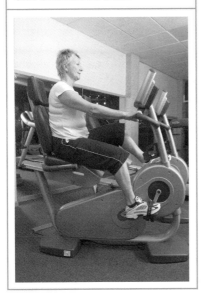

Figure 7.3 Correct position on recumbent bike

- the angle of the seat, the position of the backrest and pedals force the weight to bear down and reduce the space around the hip joint which may aggravate arthritis.
- the action at the hip during cycling on a recumbent bike pushes the weight against the hip.

Treadmill on the flat

Figure 7.4 Correct position on treadmill on the flat

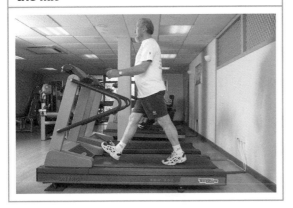

- more weight bears down on a flat surface than on an incline, creating increased joint impact.

Treadmill on an incline

Figure 7.5 Correct position on treadmill on the incline

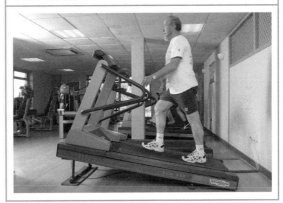

- an incline if 1–2 per cent will reduce the impact for clients with arthritis of the spine and hip.

Rowing machine

Rowing can be difficult for clients with arthritis in the knees and hips. The forward motion reduces the openness in the knee and hip joints, and weight bears slightly on the hip joint. Although if good technique is followed, and the client is interested in this form of exercise, then do not automatically rule it out. Teaching good posture is essential to avoid aggravating the condition. Be aware that rowing can also be very jarring on the neck, which is a common area for arthritis.

Figure 7.6 Correct position on rower

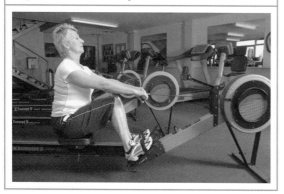

- arrows through torso indicate good posture position – long spine, shoulders dropping down away from the ears, abdominals contracted and elbows drawing in towards rib cage. Watch out for over-arching of spine and shoulders pulling forwards

Adapting and modifying resistance and hand weight exercises

The same considerations about seat position and joint action apply to weight training with a client who has arthritis. The severity of the arthritis will affect mobility, which can make it difficult to get on and off machines and aggravate an already painful condition. The following examples intend to get you to think about the movement of joints as a client gets *on and off the equipment* as well as the *joint action during the exercise.* Also included are examples of how you can progress a specific muscle group according to the ability and confidence of your client. The aim of strengthening exercises for the condition of arthritis is to maintain joint stability and diminish pain, and exercises should be performed *without load* on the affected joint, for example seated leg exercise rather than a standing squat. (see figures 7.9 and 7.10 below)

Swimming and water aerobics

If ever there was a perfect exercise for arthritis, then swimming or aqua aerobics is it, as the water supports and relieves pressure on the joints. However, using this mode of exercise will depend on how the client feels about water. Some older adults may feel self-conscious in a swimsuit and have concerns about the drying effects of chlorine on skin.

The buoyancy of water decreases the weight-bearing impact of any exercise. When submerged to shoulder level a person can experience a weight loss of 90 per cent, while at waist level the weight loss is 41 per cent (Davis and Harrison, 1988). Exercising in water will provide a client who has arthritis relief from the pressures of land-based exercise. You may need to assess how easy it is for your client to access the pool (bearing in mind potential difficulties of getting into the pool on a steep ladder and how this affects arthritic joints). Also consider that arthritis in the fingers, wrist or shoulder can reduce the amount of time a client can grip the side of the pool or any resistance equipment you use. For people with arthritis in the hip, abduction can be painful, so breaststroke arms with a paddle or flutter kick may be more comfortable. Do not recommended to clients with arthritic or problem knees. The temperature of the water and the pool area needs to be on the warmer side for people with arthritis, 84–88° F/ 29–31° C. If the water is too cold (below 87° F/ 31° C) they will feel uncomfortable and become stiff. The water must not be too hot either (over 90° F/ 32° C) as the participants could become overheated, especially if they have high blood pressure or any heart-related conditions.

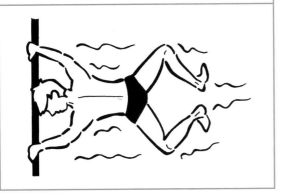

Figure 7.7 Adult in a swimming pool, holding on to the edge of the pool with legs in breast stroke position

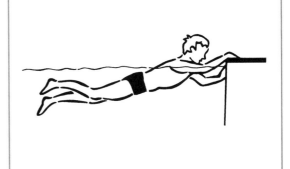

Figure 7.8 Adult in a swimming pool, holding on to the edge of the pool with legs in crawl or flutter kick position

Quadriceps and hamstring strengthening – to support the knee joint

Figure 7.9 Photograph of a seated leg extension

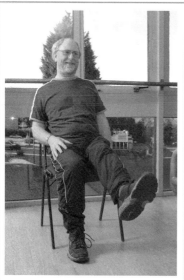

This is non-weight bearing, although be aware that there is a big stress on the knee (patella femoral joint) which can aggravate osteoarthritis. A seated chair leg extension without weights would be an alternative.

Figure 7.10 Seated leg extension adding a weight or dyna band to increase resistance

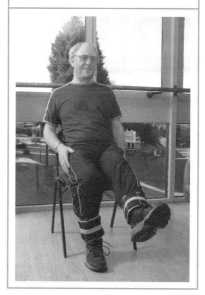

Figure 7.11 seated leg extension on resistance machine

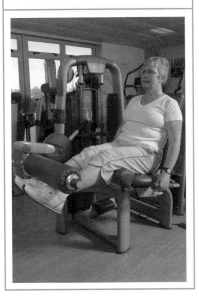

Figure 7.13 Hamstring curls holding the back of a chair

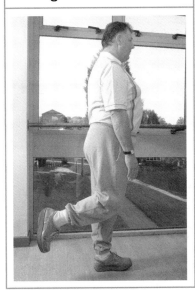

Figure 7.12 Photograph of a standing squat

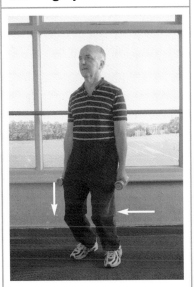

This is a weight-bearing activity. Arrows and dotted line will indicate where the weight is bearing down on the joint.

Figure 7.14 Hamstring curls holding the back of a chair or bar adding a leg weight

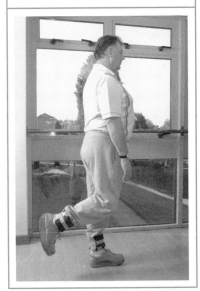

Figure 7.15 Seated leg curl

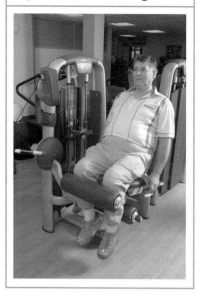

Back strengthening to support the spine, neck and shoulders

Figure 7.16 Lat pull down

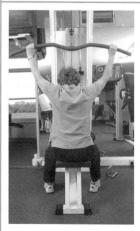
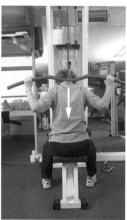

The arrows indicate how the weight bears down during the action of a lat pull down. This exercise can cause the vertebrae of the neck and spine to compress where indicated with an '↓'.

Figure 7.17 Vertical row

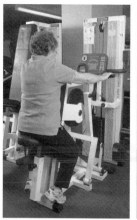
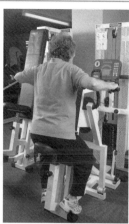

The action of this movement does not weight bear on the spine or neck.

Shoulder stability and strength

Again select exercises that are comfortable for the client. Arthritis in the shoulder and lack of use may make arm abduction difficult, and full range of movement is a goal to progress towards. It is a good idea to combine mobilisation exercises with strength work. For example, standing hip extension will mobilise the hip, seated leg extension and curl will mobilise the knee and shoulder rolls with free weights will mobilise the shoulders.

Figure 7.18 Side lateral raise position with arm held below full range of movement

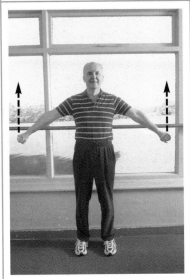

The arrows indicate a full range of movement as the aim of the exercise. Observe the range of movement and aim to increase it over time with daily mobility and stretching exercises. The extent you will be able to improve the range of movement will depend on the severity of the arthritis. Remember, when working with clients who have arthritis there will almost always be some level of pain to tolerate, so be patient and supportive of your client.

Summary

- arthritis affects the joints and causes stiffness and swelling around the joints
- arthritis has different levels of severity and can be a very painful condition
- clients should always exercise within the limitations of their pain threshold
- rest is advised for clients with rheumatoid arthritis during painful flare ups
- arthritis limits the range of movement of the joint
- avoid weight or loading the joint
- be aware of the angle of the joint throughout the range of movement and at the beginning and end phase of an action
- observe range of movement on abduction and be aware of any increases in pain
- be alert to the position of seats on equipment and how they affect the angle of the joint during the exercise
- consider ease of getting on and off the equipment
- combine mobilisation with strength work for more freedom of joint movement.

Lower back pain

What is lower back pain?

Lower back pain is one of the most common chronic pain problems in our society. Almost everyone will have at least one episode of lower back pain during his or her life. There are many ideas about what causes lower back pain, and these causes can be related to damage, normal ageing of the spine and discs, muscular problems, arthritis of the spine, problems with ligaments and tendons around the spine, poor posture and manual handling techniques.

The lumbar spine is the most vulnerable area and suffers a great amount of wear and tear compared to other parts of the spine. This is due to the greatest amount of abnormal stress being placed on the lower lumbar spine during excessive bending and twisting and adopting poor postural habits. It is often difficult to locate the source of pain because of the complex network of nerve fibres that sends messages to muscles and ligaments. The experience of pain causes physical and emotional reactions that may deter your client from exercising. However, it is important to begin or maintain aerobic, endurance, strength and flexibility during the first two weeks of the *acute phase* (less than three months) of lower back pain. An acute episode of lower back pain can be very severe, lasting for a few days or a week and then will often improve, although the length and intensity of the pain will depend on the individual and their ability to cope with pain.

Types of back pain

1. In a relatively small number of cases back pain may be caused by the compression of a 'nerve root', which is the start of a nerve as it leaves the spinal cord. It is usually caused when a vertebral disc becomes displaced from its normal position (commonly known as a *slipped disc*). However, slipped discs mainly occur in 18–30 year olds, and the cause of nerve root pain for older adults is due to the wear and tear of the spine which narrows the exit for the spinal nerve.
2. Sciatic nerve pain may result in 'referred pain' down the leg to the calves, feet and toes.
3. Clients who have back pain that lasts longer than a week should consult their GP, and if they have any of the following symptoms should consult their GP immediately:

- fever
- redness or swelling of the back
- pain down the legs and below the knees
- numbness or weakness in one or both legs
- loss of bladder control
- back pain caused by an injury, fall or blow to the back
- constant pins and needles in one or both feet.

It is generally accepted that patients with either acute or chronic lower back pain will benefit from:

- back strengthening exercises (see figures 7.20–7.33 for examples)
- stretching to encourage and restore movement of the spine and muscles
- core stability and posture training (see the perfect posture box on page 93 and the neutral spine and core activation box on page 94)
- advice on correct lifting will also help prevent your client aggravate or cause an episode of lower back pain (see lifting technique box on page 93).

Perfect posture

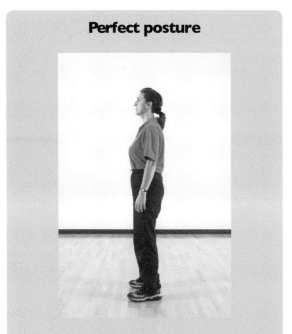

- stand with feet together or hip width apart if more comfortable
- balance your weight on all four corners of your feet
- draw the muscles of your legs inwards by tightening them upwards and sinking your feet deeper into the floor
- feel your knee caps drawing upwards
- tuck your tail bone under and gently draw it forwards
- pull your belly button back towards your spine
- widen across your mid back
- create more space between your collarbones
- slide your shoulder blades down your back
- draw your head back so that your chin does not protrude
- extend and lengthen the spine and neck upwards.

Correct lifting technique

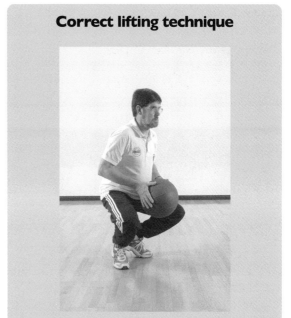

- always lift correctly and lift only a manageable weight
- think as you lift
- always keep a straight back when lifting, pushing or pulling – do not twist at the same time
- bend your knees not your back
- when picking up an object, bend your knees, face the object and pick up the object from a lowered position
- draw the bellybutton in towards the spine before you rise up
- keep the back straight as you rise up into a standing position.

Exercise recommendations

Goals

The priority is to relieve back pain as well as prevent the spiral of decline (see pages 77–8) by developing core stability, good posture and back care in lifting and daily living. Once good habits are instilled, the risk of injury in cardiovascular training and strength training is reduced. Flexibility, mobility and relaxation are also important components of this programme.

Cardiovascular training

Low impact aerobics such as treadmill walking and upright or recumbent cycling can be started at the onset of lower back pain, although be aware that certain standing and sitting positions can aggravate the pain. As part of the induction get your client to try out the different machines that are available, and identify those that minimise pain.

Strength training

Emphasise the importance of activating core stability (see the core activation box below). The main consideration is to avoid any machines or free weight exercises that compress the spine or that excessively twist the spine, for example rotary torso. It is very important that you work closely with the client to establish the difference between discomfort and pain.

Flexibility and range of movement (ROM)

All standard flexibility and ROM exercises are suitable unless they aggravate the pain. As with cardiovascular and strength training it is a case of working out what best suits your client.

Special considerations

- let your client know that they are likely to experience some discomfort and that they must inform you when they experience pain, and if it continues after cessation of exercise
- lower back pain that is unrelenting can be very stressful for your client and difficult to cope with on some days more than others, so be aware of this
- tension and stress will only increase your client's perception of the intensity of any pain they are feeling, and it would be helpful to teach them relaxation and breathing techniques outlined on pages 157–60.

Client care and education

Encourage your client to become more aware of how they lift and move the spine in daily life, and when sitting and standing (see the box on correct lifting technique on page 93).

It is very important that you work closely with the client to establish the difference between discomfort and pain.

Neutral/natural curve of the spine

- knees are soft and shoulder blades rest in a soft 'v'
- curl the pelvis forward and back as if filling and emptying a bucket of water – the fill is the pelvis coming forward and the emptying as you move back
- aim to get to the halfway point where the water in the bucket is level, which will bring the spine into neutral position.

Core activation

- place hands flatly and firmly on tummy area, thumbs touching at bellybutton
- pull navel towards the spine as you take a full and deep breath
- release fully and repeat a few times
- repeat the above and release the abdominal muscles 50 per cent, but continue to release the breath 100 per cent
- repeat until you have got the hang of it
- repeat again but this time release the abdominal muscles 70 per cent while exhaling fully
- repeat until you have a good awareness of what holding in the abdominal muscles at 70 per cent means.

Table 7.1	Three-step programme to support clients with lower back pain

1. Spend time with your client analysing their posture in front of the mirror:
- identify any poor posture signs such as rounded shoulders, slouched position, stomach jutting forwards, exaggerated lordosis of the spine or weight leaning to one side
- teach and practise perfect postural alignment with your client (see the box on page 93)
- teach neutral spine and core muscle activation (see the box on page 94).

2. Teach back strengthening exercises and relaxation techniques
(see figures 7.30–7.33 for example exercises and pages 153–5 for relaxation techniques)

3. Introduce aerobic, strength training and resistance exercises

Be aware that many older adults are uncomfortable getting up and down from the floor and many will have weak wrists, ankles and knees.

Back strengthening exercises

The following exercises will help to strengthen the muscles of the back, abdomen, hips and quadriceps and improve posture. The repetitions are guidelines only – adjust them as your client's ability dictates. Be aware of any conditions that make it difficult or painful to get into some positions.

Beginners

Figure 7.20 Wall slide

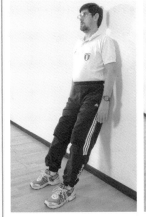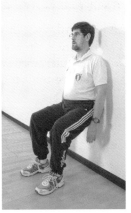

- stand with back against a wall with feet shoulder width apart
- walk feet 12 inches from wall
- keep core muscles activated while slowly bending knees to 45-degrees
- hold for five seconds and slowly slide back up
- repeat 5–10 times.

Figure 7.21 Heel slide

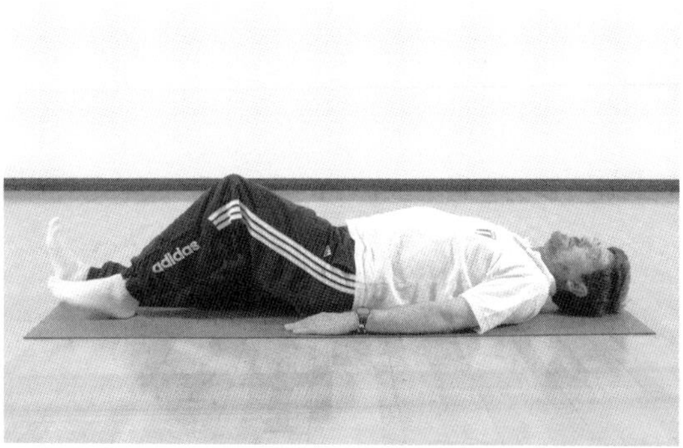

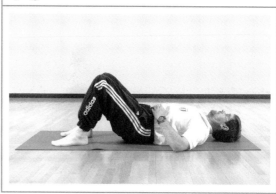

- lie on back with straight legs
- slowly slide heel along the floor, bending and straightening the leg
- repeat 5–10 times each side, alternating between legs.

Figure 7.22 Abdominal strengthener – lying flat

- lie on back with knees bent and hands below ribs
- tighten abdominal muscles and press rib cage down to meet hip, close the gap between ribs and hips
- do not hold breath, or lift head off floor
- hold for five seconds, and repeat 5–10 times.

Figure 7.25 Straight leg raises

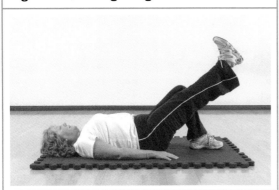

Figure 7.26 Knee to chest hug (to decrease strain on back)

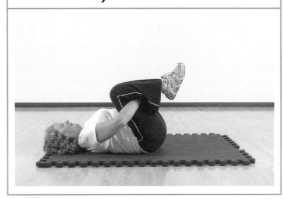

Intermediate

- lie on back with one leg straight and one leg bent
- activate core muscles to stabilise lower back
- slowly raise straight leg 6–12 inches
- hold for 1–5 seconds
- slowly lower leg
- repeat 5–10 times on each side.

- lie on floor with knees bent and feet flat on floor
- raise both knees towards chest and place hands under knees
- hug knees as close to chest as possible for 1–5 seconds
- keep head and shoulders on floor
- lower legs, keeping knees bent
- repeat 5–10 times.

Figure 7.27 Leg raises with chair option

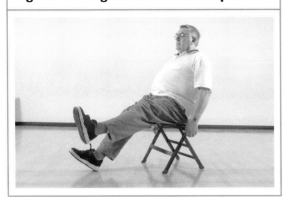

- sit in upright chair with back support
- extend and straighten legs with heels resting on the floor
- lift one leg to waist height, gently pushing the heel forwards, and hold for 10 seconds
- slowly return leg to the floor
- repeat 5–10 times on each side.

Figure 7.28 Lumber stabilisation with swiss ball

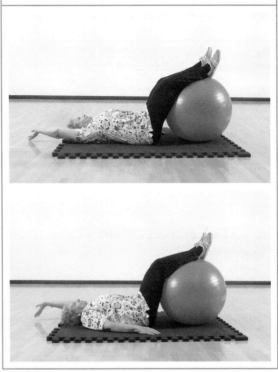

- core muscles must remain activated for this exercise to be effective
- lie on your back with knees bent and calves resting on a ball
- slowly raise arm over head and lower arms, alternating between the right and left side
- slowly straighten one knee and relax, alternating between the right and left side
- slowly straighten one knee and raise opposite arm over head, alternating opposite arms and legs
- slowly walk ball forwards and backwards with legs.

Advanced

Figure 7.29 Hip flexor stretch

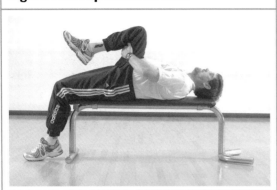

Figure 7.30 Periformis stretch

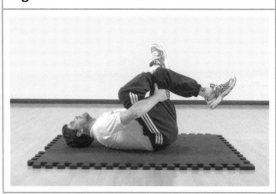

- lie on back near edge of either bed or bench
- hold knee to chest
- slowly lower one leg down, keeping the knee bent until a stretch can be felt across top of the hip/thigh and hold for 20 seconds
- repeat 5 times on each side.

- lie on back with both knees bent
- cross one leg over the other and pull knee of lower leg to chest until a stretch can be felt
- hold for 20 seconds and relax
- repeat 5 times on each side.

Figure 7.31 Core stability and swiss ball

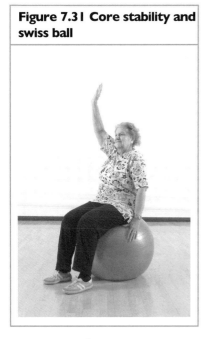

- core muscle must remain activated for this exercise to be effective
- slowly raise arm overhead and then lower arm, alternating right and left sides
- slowly raise and lower heel, alternating right and left sides
- slowly raise one heel and raise opposite arm overhead. Alternate opposite arms and heels
- marching – slowly raise one foot 2 inches from floor, alternating right and left sides.

Summary

- it is important to remain active and mobile with back pain unless symptoms outlined under 'types of back pain' indicate otherwise
- exercise should be low impact
- good posture and core stability are a priority for back care
- core stability will improve posture and help recovery from injury and lower back pain
- back pain in older adults can be caused by:
    - ageing of discs
    - muscular problems
    - arthritis of the spine
    - problems with ligaments and tendons around the spine
    - displaced vertebrae.

Anne's case study

I have always been active – in my teens I cycled every day and belonged to an athletics club where I did running and discus. I also rode horses, and practised ballroom and Latin dancing to teacher level.

I was married at 22 and had three sons in fairly quick succession. The first time I experienced any knee pain was when my husband and I took up hill walking, and I was coming down a steep incline. When on level ground or climbing uphill there wasn't a problem. It gradually wore off, and although I had twinges every so often it was nothing serious.

At 26 I started playing squash, and would often be playing five times a week at a reasonable level. For many years my knees behaved themselves, although I was always conscious I needed to warm them up thoroughly. However, gradually I began to get pain in my left knee again. I eventually had an arthroscopy* in 1996. This was successful and I carried on playing, although I did play a little less.

In 2004 I experienced another increase in pain and difficulty in moving – squash demands speed and agility, and mine seemed to be disappearing. My surgeon said there was more cartilage degeneration, but wasn't considering any further surgery. In the end I had to give up playing squash.

I then needed to find another way of retaining my fitness and mobility. I started playing racket ball once a week (similar to squash but not so demanding on the legs). I also did classes in 'Body Pump' for strength and 'Body Balance' for suppleness and flexibility, spent an hour in the gym once a week for a cardiovascular workout, and walked once or twice a week between 7–12 miles. In all the classes I have adapted and modified to what I can do, and omit what I can't to avoid further stress and pain, keeping my knee joint mobile.

Sometimes it would be easy to miss out exercise – but I don't. It takes self-discipline, but the results are worth the effort. I think of it like a car, you keep that serviced regularly. More exercise results in more energy. There is no point in doing something you don't enjoy, but it helps to keep the activities numerous and varied. Everyone will experience some physical difficulties as the years advance, and I prefer to work around them and do more than I think I can – a positive mental attitude is vital.

*Arthroscopy is an inspection of the joint cavity with an arthroscope enabling surgical removal of the cartilage.

Osteoporosis

Osteoporosis is a condition that makes bones very vulnerable to the risk of bone fracture, even under minimum stress. Actions as simple as bending and lifting or a very slight knock can cause a bone fracture. Everyone over the age of 35 starts to lose a minute amount of bone mass each year. For some this also combines with a loss of lean body mass and an inactive lifestyle, leading to 1 in 2 women and 1 in 8 men over the age of 50 having an osteoporotic hip fracture.

Osteoporosis can be a disabling and painful condition that limits mobility, and can cause a great deal of psychological distress to the sufferer. The main consideration when developing an exercise programme for a client who has osteoporosis is to establish the severity of the condition. The symptoms of osteoporosis can go undetected for some time, and usually begin to show around the ages of 60–70. As bones lose their mineral content the thoracic region of the spine curves over and kyphosis of the spine develops (see the Back to Basics box below). However, it is more likely that you will be working with clients on a preventative level or with the aim of minimising deterioration. The programme should include weight bearing activity and resistance training with specific exercises that focus on improving balance.

What is osteoporosis?

Osteoporosis is a loss of bone mineral density that causes bones to become brittle and highly susceptible to fracture – particularly in the hip, spine and wrists. One of the major factors contributing to osteoporosis includes the decline of bone mass associated with ageing, which increases in women during menopause. Other lifestyle factors that affect bone density are smoking, excessive alcohol intake, poor

Back basics

- Kyphosis is an exaggerated curve of the spine (more commonly known as hunchback). Kyphosis may be caused by degeneration of the intervertebral discs, poor posture and rickets (bones that do not harden in childhood due to a Vitamin D deficiency). It is also common in women with advanced osteoporosis. The term 'round shoulders' is an expression for mild Kyphosis.
- Lordosis is an exaggerated curve of the lumbar spine and can be caused by obesity, weight gain of the abdomen (in pregnancy, for example), poor posture, rickets, and tuberculosis of the spine.

nutrition and lack of physical activity. As a result of a decline in activity of bone forming cells, all human beings over the age of 35 lose a minute amount of bone mass each year. Women are at a higher risk as they may experience a 3–5 year acceleration of bone loss after menopause due to a loss of oestrogen. Men are less likely to experience bone loss before the age of 70 unless other lifestyle factors, diseases or medications cause a loss of bone mass or strength.

If your client experiences pain, avoid exercises over or near the spine and any exercises that involve back extension or forward flexion, for example bent over row or weight machines such as abdominal or back extension machines.

Clients with osteoporosis may have hairline fractures and are very vulnerable to bone fractures, which makes core stability, posture and balance exercises an important element of the exercise programme.

Exercise recommendations

Goals

To improve or maintain aerobic fitness, strength and posture; to improve core stability and balance and reduce the risk of falls.

Cardiovascular training

All modes of exercise are possible, although avoid twisting the spine at all times. You may want to avoid rowing machines due to the forward flexion movement, unless core stability is developed enough to retain good posture and technique. Weight bearing aerobic exercise has been shown to be beneficial for slowing osteoporosis, and can lead to improvements in the density of the bone receiving the load and muscle force.

Strength training

It is advisable to progress through the resistance programme slowly. Start with light resistance bands, progress to free weights and then to resistance machines. *The American College of Sports Medicine* recommends that the best results are achieved when clients can progress to relatively high weights with fewer repetitions (75 per cent of 1RM). Include postural exercises that will improve or prevent rounding of the shoulders and upper back.

Flexibility and range of movement

Stretching and joint mobilisation should be done daily, although avoid twisting or forward flexion of the spine. Kyphosis of the spine can result in the chest and neck muscles becoming tight, so focus on exercises and stretches that retract the shoulder blade (see modifications and adaptations on pages 104–5). Include hip flexor stretches as they can become tight as a result of ageing, and from walking with poor or stooped posture.

Special considerations

- ensure that the exercise environment is safe with minimal obstacles and stable flooring to reduce the risk and anxiety of falling. Be aware of any slight changes in level from stretch mat to hard floor or hidden steps
- if your client has pain, avoid exercise near or over the spine
- balance training combined with strength training will help reduce risk of falls.

Client care and education

- regular exercise can slow the age-related loss of bone mass
- good strength, posture and balance all reduce the risk of falls
- strength training of both the upper and lower body will maximise benefits
- use correct technique for all exercises
- avoid excessive forward flexion of the spine, which can cause fractures and place internal organs in a vulnerable position leading to injury
- avoid hyperextension of the spine as it can contribute to spinal fractures
- avoid ballistic or jarring movements
- practise balance activities only when support is available
- avoid standing on one leg for extended periods, which may place vulnerable hips at risk
- avoid activities with a high risk of falling.

Risk factors for osteoporosis

- female
- advanced age
- white/asian
- family history of osteoporosis
- low body weight for height
- premature menopause
- low testosterone levels in men
- lack of physical activity
- heavy smoking
- excessive alcohol consumption
- low dietary calcium intake
- chronic use of medications causing bone loss

In addition to pain, a client with osteoporosis may be anxious about falling. Create a range of physical supports throughout the programme and identify clear pathways during transitions to other areas in the gym. Make your client aware of any high risk fall areas such as a step or loose mats, and free weights areas where weights may be left on the floor.

Exercise modifications for clients with osteoporosis

As for clients with arthritis, think about what is happening to the spine during an exercise. The equipment and exercises you select should be based on your awareness of how the mechanics of the exercise will affect the spine. Focus on exercises that retract the shoulder blades.

Avoid the following exercises if your client has osteoporosis

- back extension and back flexion exercises
- bent over row
- overhead press and lat pull down
- resistance machines that need spinal flexion
- abdominal machines
- back extension machines

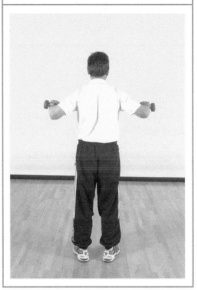

Figure 7.35 Shoulder retraction machines/weights

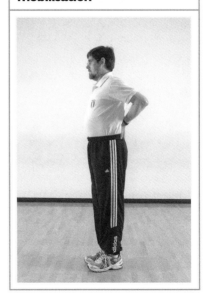

Figure 7.36 Chest stretch for daily stretching and joint mobilisation

Bill's case study

Despite having kidney problems since the age of 11, I have always been active. I lost my twin brother at the age 9 because of kidney problems, and when I was 50 I suffered from kidney failure, and underwent a transplant. I had to take 10 weeks off work, but my recovery went well – two weeks after the operation I kept myself busy around the home painting and decorating. In the long term the kidney transplant means that I have to take immune suppressant drugs that stop my body rejecting the kidney. The drugs work by breaking down the immune system, leaving me susceptible to colds and viruses. They have also caused me to have 'drug induced diabetes' which is something I have to manage.

During my recovery time following the transplant, I started an exercise programme at the hospital that consisted of a circuit of aerobic and strength exercises. After I went back to work it became difficult for me to get there, and so the diabetic nurse told me about the GP referral scheme at Harlow Sportcentre which was much more convenient.

In September 2004 I started out with a 12-minute aerobic programme at a low intensity that included:

- treadmill (3 minutes)
- upright cycle (3 minutes)

- rotex (1 minute)
- recumbent cycle (2 minutes)
- treadmill (3 minutes)

By August 2005 my aerobic training had increased to 1 hour 14 minutes, and I have progressed the intensity, speed and resistance on each of them. I also include some resistance machines such as chest press, vertical press, abductor and adductor machine for improving my upper and lower body strength.

I started out very slowly and gradually built up the programme. I am now a full member of the gym having completed the 10-week GP referral scheme. I train four times a week and then play golf once a week. The social side of the gym is also good for me – because I work as a taxi driver in London it can be quite isolating. I have met some interesting people at the gym and made some new friends. As a taxi driver approaching 60 I have to take a fitness test and Marion, my fitness instructor, is looking into the pass criteria. I know I will be ready for it because physically I feel I am in good shape – I have increased stamina and strength, and my breathing is a lot easier. Going to the gym is a priority for me now, and it comes before anything else. I have also learnt how to manage my diabetes and if I have any questions I only have to ask the instructors.

Table 7.2	At a glance exercise programming for musculoskeletal conditions			
Condition/ mode	Cardiovascular training	Strength training	Flexibility and range of movement	Additional advice
Arthritis	Low impact non-weight bearing: Walking; cycling; rowing; swimming; dance; aqua aerobics (water temperature 85–90° F or 29–32° C.)	Circuit training, free weights, bands, isometric exercises (if no other contraindication is present such as hypertension and coronary heart disease).	Passive stretching, active stretching	Cross train to avoid overuse of certain joints. Minimise pain with ice and heat treatment before and after exercise. Advise client to wear good supporting shoes with shock absorbing insoles.
Intensity/duration	Build from 5–30 minutes, 5 times a week.	2–3 reps building up to 10–12 reps, 2–3 days a week.	1–2 times daily.	Warm up and cool down are especially important for people with arthritis because of joint stiffness.
Goal	60–80 per cent of HR max. RPE 11–15. Focus progression on duration over intensity.	Increase muscle strength to support and stabilise joint. Low reps initially. Emphasis on hip flexors and extensors, back extensors and lower abdominals.	Increase and maintain pain free ROM. Reduce stiffness.	
Osteoporosis	Walking, cycling, swimming and aqua aerobics	Free weights, resistance machines, ankle and wrist weights, body resistance. Slow progression starting with resistance bands, progressing to free weights and then to resistant machines.	Passive and active stretching, chair based exercises.	
Intensity/duration	20–30mins 3–5 x a week.	2–3 days for 20–40 minutes.		Avoid excessive flexion or extension
Goal	40–70 per cent HR max. RPE 11–15.	75 per cent of 1RM. 3–10 reps.	5–7 days a week.	The emphasis is on core strength and posture improvement as a falls prevention strategy. Include balance exercises with support.

Table 7.2	At a glance exercise programming for musculoskeletal conditions cont.			
Condition/ mode	Cardiovascular training	Strength training	Flexibility and range of movement	Additional advice
Lower back pain	Walking, cycling upright or recumbent if pain is manageable.	Core stability exercises, abdominal and back extensor strengthening, pelvic floor exercises	Head to toe flexibility and mobility daily.	Avoid high impact exercises and excessive rotation and twisting of spine. Avoid back and hip exercises during first two weeks of flare up.
Intensity/duration	Low–moderate intensity.	10–20 reps. Increase reps as tolerated.	Hold each stretch for 10 seconds	Teach correct lifting technique and posture awareness.
Goal	40–70 per cent HR max. RPE 11–15. Maintain or improve CV fitness.	Back strengthening exercises daily. Improve abdominal and lower back strength.	Increase and maintain pain-free flexibility and ROM	

Further reading

Durstine, L. J. and Moore, G. E. (2003) *ACSM's Exercise Management for Persons with Chronic Diseases and Disabilities* (Human Kinetics)

Egger, G. and Champion, N. (1990) *The Fitness Leaders Handbook*, third edition (A&C Black)

Jessie Jones, C. and Rose, Debra J. (2005), *Physical Activity Instruction of Older Adults* (Human Kinetics)

Oxford Concise Medical Dictionary (2003, Oxford University Press)

Poggiali, T. and Peters, K. (2000) *Step in the Right Direction Manual* (Keiser Institute on Ageing)

Tortora, G. J. and Grabowski, S. R. (1993) *Principles of Anatomy and Physiology*, seventh edition (HarperCollins)

Online resources

www.americanheart.org
www.backcare.org.uk
www.britishpainsocieity.org
www.helptheaged.org.uk
www.wrightfoundation.com, for information on medically led exercise referral programme qualifications.

Jane's case study

During the night I had awoken with a start at 4.30 am. I felt fine apart from a small ache in my left armpit – I tried to get back to sleep but couldn't. After another hour spent tossing and turning, I began to feel strange. Suddenly I had to rush to the bathroom and I was violently sick. My tummy began to ache too, and I had an upset stomach. I felt hot and sweaty. After a while I went downstairs and decided to phone the duty doctor, who, after a lot of questions, told me to call an ambulance.

The paramedics didn't seem anxious. On arrival at hospital I was given lots of tests, but still had no pain at all. Suddenly a doctor and several nurses rushed to my bed, 'you're having a heart attack' the doctor said me, 'I need your permission to give you a clot-busting drug, but I do have to tell you it may cause you to have a stroke'. I felt numb with shock and paralysed with fear. This can't be right – they must have made a mistake. After all I was a fairly young looking 52 year old woman, and had never really had any health concerns.

The next day I was totally numb with shock. I kept asking 'why me?' – I had always exercised and I had a good diet. I felt so scared, alone and reluctant to move in case it happened again! I felt convinced that my life was over. As the long and difficult process of rehabilitation began I found that I couldn't stand to be on my own, and I was scared to go to sleep. I was a total wreck and could not believe that I had changed so much in such a short time. Three weeks later a letter arrived inviting me to a Phase 3 rehabilitation class at the hospital – I looked forward to this with some trepidation.

The classes were interesting and most informative, and the nurses were reassuring and endlessly patient with me. Although I found the classes emotionally and physically demanding I persevered, and my confidence increased. After a month I transferred to a Phase 4 class, which I found was different to the Phase 3 class. Afterwards we met for tea and a chat – people were laughing and telling jokes! It was fun!

Everyone's story was different and interesting. When I found out that some of the participants had been coming for 1–2 years I began to see that life could go on.

I really began to look forward to the class. The staff were wonderful – they answered questions and addressed any worries and they made the class fun. The actual exercise was great and we worked very hard. The friendships I have formed are mutually supportive and rewarding – we have a natural affinity with each other evolving from our experiences.

I have now been attending rehab classes for about eighteen months in total, and I really love it. Most of the time I feel back to normal, although I can still get very tired. Unfortunately, however, not many women attend rehab classes – maybe this is due to family pressures, looking after grandchildren, work demands or the stigma attached as heart disease is still considered to be primarily a male disease. In fact, heart disease is the biggest killer of *both* men *and* women in the developed world.

My life has changed irrevocably over the last eighteen months, and I know that it will never be the same again. I have learnt to listen to my body and to trust my intuition. Just like everyone else who has had a heart attack, I have good and bad days – and what happened to me is never far from my mind. However, I know that I wouldn't be where I am today without the support that I received from family and friends, and above all from the rehab classes – 'The Club'!

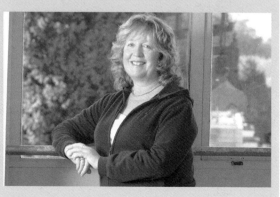

DIABETES

8

Physical activity is important for people with diabetes, and is a central component of diabetes treatment. People who have diabetes have an increased risk of cardiovascular disease, which has been attributed in part to a sedentary lifestyle, and in part to the fact that 80–90 per cent of people with type II diabetes are overweight or obese. Regular exercise can help diabetics stabilise their blood sugar levels, control their weight, reduce the risk of cardiovascular disease and also have a significant impact on reducing body weight. A combination of exercise, diet and regulation of blood glucose levels will help to manage diabetes.

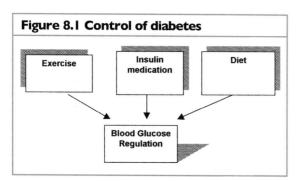

Figure 8.1 Control of diabetes

Research has shown that increased physical activity in conjunction with dietary changes can prevent those who are insulin resistant progressing to type II diabetes.

What is Diabetes?

Diabetes is a metabolic disorder where the pancreas is unable to produce or effectively utilise insulin and therefore unable to control sugar levels in the blood (blood glucose levels).

Insulin is required for converting glucose into energy in the blood cells

There are two types of diabetes:

- **Type I** means that the body is unable to produce insulin, and injections or other medication is required. A GP or nurse will decide the amount of insulin and the number of injections needed. Some people may take their insulin by either a syringe or pump into different parts of the body. Type I diabetes can occur at any age, but usually before the age of 30. Exercise sessions for those who are insulin dependent may be relatively short, but higher in frequency.
- **Type II** means that the body produces some insulin but does not respond effectively, and high levels of glucose remain in the body. 80 per cent of people with type II diabetes are either overweight or obese. Treatment for this type of diabetes may consist of advice on healthy eating and increasing activity. More frequently people with type II diabetes are being prescribed insulin as it is now considered a treatment that will help control glucose levels for type II diabetics.

If you have clients who have type I diabetes and are taking insulin or other medication, you need to be aware of hypoglycaemia and hyperglycaemia, and how these conditions are affected by exercise.

- **hypoglycaemia** is a deficiency of glucose in the bloodstream caused by insulin overdose and insufficient intake of carbohydrates. Causes muscular weakness, confusion and lack of coordination and sweating.

- **hyperglycaemia** is an excess of glucose in the bloodstream due to insufficient insulin, and excessive intake of carbohydrates (see table 8.1 below).

Each client will be different, and it is important to carefully monitor how different activities and the time of day affects blood glucose levels. There will be some trial and error involved in establishing consistent habits that balance the effect of medication, diet and exercise on blood sugar levels and minimise the risk of a hypoglycaemic or hyperglycaemic attack – hypoglycaemia can occur after prolonged exercise when the body is unable to produce enough insulin to satisfy muscular demand.

Ketoacidosis

This is a condition that develops when the body does not have enough insulin. Without insulin the body cannot use glucose for fuel, so instead it breaks body fats to use for energy, producing waste products called ketones. The body cannot tolerate large amounts of ketones, and a build up will lead to ketoacidosis or a 'diabetic coma' (as it is more commonly known).

Exercise recommendations

Goal

Regular physical activity is an important part of diabetes management. The main goals are weight loss, a reduction in insulin resistance and

Table 8.1	Hypoglycaemia and hyperglycaemia – symptoms and causes
What is hypoglycaemia?	*What is hyperglycaemia?*
A deficiency of glucose in the bloodstream, caused by insulin overdose and/or insufficient intake of carbohydrates.	An excess of glucose in the bloodstream due to insufficient insulin.
Symptoms include: • grey pallor • excessive sweating • shakes • palpitations • hunger • headache • blurred vision • tingling lips or fingers • anxiety or bad temper.	*Symptoms include:* • high blood glucose • increased need to urinate • increased thirst • shortness of breath • breath that smells fruity • nausea and vomiting • can lead to a diabetic coma, a condition called *ketoacidosis* (see box above).
Causes of hypoglycaemia • too little carbohydrate • too much exercise • a change of sight for insulin injection • too much insulin • hot weather.	*Causes of hyperglycaemia* • mismanagement of medication, diet and exercise • may be triggered by infection or medications that affect glucose tolerance.

a reduction in the risks associated with coronary heart disease and high blood pressure.

Regular physical activity has many beneficial effects for patients with diabetes, and can help diabetic patients to lead normal and healthier lives. You must first establish if your client's diabetes is stable and controlled, which can be done by monitoring glucose levels before, during, and after exercise. You can also encourage your client to identify an optimal training time when glucose levels are at their most stable and read between 6–9 mmo/1.

Cardiovascular training

Cardiovascular training is recommended daily, unless other conditions such as coronary heart disease, arthritis, foot problems or blood glucose levels indicate otherwise. A low to moderate intensity of either 60–75 per cent HR max, or an RPE of 11–15 is recommended. Gradually extend the duration of exercise, building up to continuous training of at least 30 minutes. Suggest low impact or seated aerobic activities such as rowing, cycling or walking for clients who have complications with their eyes, or feet problems (see table 8.2 below).

Special considerations and screening guidelines

When managing clients with diabetes, you will need to consider the following factors:

- establish if your client's diabetes is stable and controlled and support them in trying to manage diet and exercise with their medication
- blood glucose levels should be monitored before and after activity – if the activity continues for longer than an hour then check glucose levels during activity. A glucometer can be used to monitor glucose levels before and after exercise
- type I diabetics should eat 15–30mg of carbohydrates for every 30 minutes of intense exercise
- hypoglycaemia can occur as the muscles refuel up to 36 hours after exercise.

Table 8.2	Other conditions associated with diabetes to be considered when screening

Neuropathy is damage to the nerves that sends messages from the brain and spinal cord to the muscles, skin and other parts of the body and can affect nerves that control the internal organs (autonomic nerves), motor nerves, and most commonly affects the sensory nerves of the feet and legs. Neuropathy can cause:
- pain or feelings of numbness or pins and needles in the legs
- a lack of sensation in the feet that can lead to foot ulcers that your client is unaware of so they should check their feet daily – well fitting and supportive trainers are highly recommended.

Retinopathy is caused by capillary damage in eyes. Diabetics can experience blurred vision caused by higher blood sugar levels, and are at risk of permanent damage if their blood glucose and blood pressure are not kept under control. Diabetic retinopathy is the major cause of blindness in the 30–65 age group in the UK.

Coronary Heart Disease and **high blood pressure**. Diabetics are two to three times more at risk of both these conditions – see pages 126–30 and 131–4 for more information on this.

Peripheral vascular disease is a condition that affects the blood vessels outside of the heart, in particular the legs and feet, and can cause:
- pain in legs and feet
- infections or ulcers in legs and feet
- poor wound healing.

Client care and education

- drink plenty of water as dehydration can affect blood glucose levels
- insulin injection sites should be away from muscle groups used during exercise
- consume a carbohydrate snack after exercise
- after injecting insulin avoid exercise for one hour
- wear well fitting and supportive trainers
- reassure your client that it is a normal response to breath faster and for muscles to tighten when being physically active. Clients who have previously been very sedentary may be concerned that they are harming themselves.

Work out activity goals for your client to achieve on days they do not come into the gym, for example encourage the use of a pedometer and decide with your client the number of steps that is achievable daily.

Summary

- there are two types of diabetes – insulin dependent and non-insulin dependent
- clients with diabetes are at risk of hypoglycaemia and hyperglycaemia
- people with diabetes have an increased risk of coronary heart disease, high blood pressure and peripheral vascular disease
- other conditions that are associated with diabetes are retinopathy (which can impair vision) and neuropathy (a disease of the nerves that can affect the feeling in the feet of diabetics)
- establish an optimal time for exercise when blood sugars are at their most stable.

Table 8.3	What to do if your client has a hypoglycaemic attack	
Symptoms	Step 1: raise blood sugars quickly	Step 2: prevent blood sugars falling again
<ul><li>grey pallor</li><li>excessive sweating</li><li>shakes</li><li>palpitations</li><li>hunger</li><li>headache</li><li>blurred vision</li><li>tingling lips or fingers</li><li>anxiety or bad temper.</li></ul>	Get your client to take quick-acting carbohydrates:<ul><li>3 glucose tablets or</li><li>50 ml sport energy drink or</li><li>½ glass lemonade or coke or</li><li>5 soft sweets such as fruit pastilles.</li></ul>	Get your client to take slow-acting carbohydrates:<ul><li>biscuit or</li><li>sandwich or</li><li>glass of milk or</li><li>fruit or</li><li>a meal if due.</li></ul>

NB: Recovery should take approximately 10–15 minutes.
If your client becomes unconscious, place in recovery position and dial 999.

Table 8.4	Exercise summary for diabetes			
Condition/mode	Cardiovascular training	Strength training	Flexibility and range of movement	Additional advice
Diabetes	Interval training incorporating active rest – see page 111. Walking, cycling, swimming, aqua aerobics, row, cross trainer and any large muscle activity.	Free weights, weight machines, cable and pulley systems, balance training	Passive and active stretching, yoga, Tai Chi.	Check for contra-indications such as elevated blood pressure and blood sugar levels before exercise. Gradually increase intensity, frequency and duration
Intensity/duration	4–7 days a week gradually progressing to continuous training of 30–60 minutes duration.	Low resistance/high reps.	Daily ROM and stretching of all major muscle groups.	Exercise duration for insulin-dependent diabetics should be shorter and of higher frequency.
Goal	Increase aerobic capacity 50–80 per cent HR max. RPE 11–15. Reduce CV risk factors – weight loss and unstable blood glucose levels.		Improve flexibility and range of movement.	

Further reading

Durstine, L. J. and Moore, G. E. (2003) *ACSM's Exercise Management for Persons with Chronic Diseases and Disabilities* (Human Kinetics)

Jessie Jones, C. and Rose, Debra J. (2005), *Physical Activity Instruction of Older Adults* (Human Kinetics)

Poggiali, T. and Peters, K. (2000) *Step in the Right Direction Manual* (Keiser Institute on Ageing)

Oxford Concise Medical Dictionary (2003, Oxford University Press)

Online resources

www.diabetes.org.uk
www.diabetes-healthnet.ac.uk

STROKE

9

Each year over 130,000 people in England and Wales have a stroke. Of all the people who suffer from a stroke, about a third are likely to die within the first 10 days, about a third are likely to make a recovery within one month and about a third are likely to be left disabled and needing rehabilitation.

Stroke has a greater disability impact than any other medical condition. A quarter of a million people are living with long-term disability as a result of stroke in the UK.

Like coronary obstructive pulmonary disease and chronic heart disease, the rehabilitation of stroke patients initially needs the knowledge and understanding of specialist physiotherapists. They are unlikely to seek a fitness instructor's advice unless you make connections through a hospital rehabilitation programme. Working in partnership with a physiotherapist to develop a safe and effective exercise programme is highly recommended, and will ensure that the correct technique and progression of exercise is not compromised for speed and stamina gains. A stroke can cause paralysis of limbs or specific muscles and can affect one complete side of the body. The progression of the exercise programme will be guided by the mobility and strength of the weaker side to avoid compensation of the stronger side. Training people who have had a stroke requires patience and a willingness to provide emotional and physical support. It involves retraining clients in the basic mechanics of moving and reactivating muscles that have been weakened as a result of a stroke. For instructors the progress may appear very slow, and it will take a particularly patient trainer to be successful with a client who has had a stroke. However, persistence *will* get results, leading to an improved quality of life for the stroke patience, and a deep sense of satisfaction for the instructor.

What is a stroke?

The majority of strokes happen when a blood clot blocks one of the arteries that carry blood to the brain. This deprives the brain cells of the oxygen they need, which causes that area to become damaged or even die. A stroke is a neuromuscular disorder that is medically referred to as a cerebrovascular accident (CVA), and can be caused by either:

1. a thrombus (blood clot) which results in sudden decrease of blood flow to the brain which is medically referred to as an 'ischaemic stroke' (ischemia means an inadequate flow of blood.)
2. a haemorrhage or 'haemorrhagic stroke' is caused by a leaking or ruptured blood cells in and around the arteries causing bleeding in or around the brain.

The symptoms of stroke and the extent to which they will affect a person will depend on which part of the brain is affected by the stroke, the severity of the stroke and the person's age and level of fitness. Common symptoms of stroke include:

- numbness
- weakness or paralysis affecting one side of the body, or an arm or leg, or one side of the face.

The outcome of a stroke results in an impairment of the central nervous system causing a loss of motor and sensory function in the legs and arms, or down one side. A stroke can also:

- affect speech ability
- cause mental confusion
- affect field of vision
- cause a condition called *apraxia*, resulting in disjointed movement.

Depending on the severity of the stroke, clients may have muscle weakness and a limited range of motion. They may also have difficulty balancing, and need assistance during their session. When writing an exercise programme for stroke clients, also refer to the guidelines for hypertension. Hypertension is a major risk for a secondary stroke, and stroke patients also have a greater risk of coronary heart disease.

Exercise recommendations

Goals

To improve the quality of life, the client's ability to carry out activities for daily living (see page 117) and regain some independence. To improve mobility and motor function. To prevent the spiral of decline (see page 78) and decrease risk of secondary stroke or cardiovascular disease. Improve aerobic fitness and static and dynamic balance.

Cardiovascular training

The debilitating motor effects of a stroke make ordinary movements take more effort and require twice the energy than would be needed by an able-bodied person. Your recommendations will be guided by the level of ability to exercise, which will depend on the severity of the stroke and your client's balance. CV training can include cycling, walking on a treadmill, step climbing or rowing and will often require some level of assistance. The intensity will depend on your client's level of fitness and, if appropriate, start with 40 per cent HR max building up to 70 per cent HR max (or at a RPE of 11–15). You may need to take an accumulative approach and build up the duration of exercise between 'active rest' using interval training (see page 40). Research has shown that patients in hospital who participate in simple exercise such as repeated sitting to standing reduce their deterioration, and improve their ability to cope with exercise.

Strength training

Strength training is important for stroke clients, as they are likely to have less functional muscle mass resulting in a weakness on one side of the body. You may have to start resistance exercises in a seated position, and simple side arm raises without any weights may be all a stroke client can achieve initially. You may have to begin strength training using their body resistance and isometric exercise, progressing to free weights or wrist and ankle weights and then onto resistance machines. You may also have to adapt the positions for carrying out resistance exercises to compensate for loss of balance. Include appropriate resistance exercises for core and leg strength as part of balance training.

Flexibility and ROM

Gradually increase range of movement of affected limbs and include stretches after strength work.

Special considerations

- arthritis is common with clients who have had a stroke
- there is an increased risk of cardiovascular disease and peripheral artery disease

- exercise equipment may have to be modified, for example strapping arms or feet to equipment
- heart rate may be lower because of medication
- a stroke can affect ability to follow instruction and may affect behaviour
- the psychological and emotional effects of a stroke require extra sensitivity and care from the trainer
- maintaining balance requires the normal functioning of many parts of the brain which can be affected by stroke. To maintain balance, nerve messages travel from the ear to the brain and to a part of the brain called the cerebellum. The cerebellum, which is situated at the base of the brain, is sometimes affected by stroke.
- stroke can also affect the parts of the brain that control eyesight. The most common problem with eyesight after stroke is the loss of one half of the field of vision where everything over to one side can be seen and there is blindness on the other side. As with other problems after a stroke, the majority of patients recover.

Client care and education

After a stroke there is greater risk of another occurring. Other lifestyle changes that can reduce the risk are:

- **diet** – a healthy diet can reduce the risk of stroke, and diets low in cholesterol and salt can help keep blood pressure within normal limits, and prevent the build-up of fatty deposits in the wall of the arteries.
- **drug therapy to prevent blood clots** – some people may be advised to take drugs to reduce the risk of blood clots forming and causing stroke. Aspirin has probably saved more lives by preventing stroke and heart attacks than any other drug. New drugs to prevent clots are now also available. Some people may also be advised to take an anticoagulant such as *Warfarin*.
- **exercise** – exercise after stroke is important for maintaining physical fitness and maximising function and can reduce the risk of further stroke. It will also help to control blood pressure, weight and cholesterol, thereby reducing the risk of further stroke.
- **lowering blood pressure** – high blood pressure is the most important risk factor for stroke. Keeping blood pressure within normal limits is essential to both prevent a stroke and reduce the risk of recurrence.

Mini strokes are when blood flow to the brain is only briefly interrupted; the symptoms are similar to stroke but last less than 24 hours, and there is always a complete recovery.

Table 9.1	Exercise summary for stroke			
Condition/mode	Cadiovascular training	Strength training	Flexibility	Additional advice
Stroke	Upper and lower body; ergometer upright cycle or recumbent cycle, seated stepper or treadmill.	Weight machines, free weights, bands or cuff weights. Own body weight as resistance.	Passive or active stretches in upper and lower body, emphasising the affected side of the body.	Use equipment with a supportive back rest if balance is unstable.
Intensity/duration	40–70 per cent of HR max or RPE 13–15, 3–5 times a week for 20–60 minutes.	3 x 8–12 reps twice a week.	At every session – before exercise, after CV component, between strength exercises and at the end of the session. Hold for 15–30 seconds.	Be aware of balance limitations and modify positions, i.e. perform resistance exercises in a seated position or while holding onto a support.
Goal	Increase speed and distance	Strengthen areas of muscle weakness, improve posture and stabilise balance.	Increase range of movement.	Balance and mobility training will reduce the risk of falls.

CHRONIC OBSTRUCTIVE PULMONARY DISEASE (COPD)

10

People who have COPD require specialist advice and support. They are unlikely to seek a fitness professional's advice unless you make connection through a hospital rehabilitation programme or a local support group. If you are interested in training clients with COPD you can identify local 'breathe easy' support groups by contacting the British Lung Foundation (see online resources on page 125). An exercise project specifically aimed at COPD clients for BACR or level 3 qualified instructors was launched during 2005, and piloted at 10 breathe easy groups nationally. There are over 150 breathe easy groups in the UK, and this could be an opportunity for fitness professionals who are interested in developing their professional skills and working with specialist populations.

You will need to have empathy with your client as COPD can be a very frightening disease. Imagine the panic and stress you would feel if you were not able to get enough oxygen to breathe properly all day, every day, seven days a week.

During rehabilitation, an oximeter is used to check the oxygen saturation of the client during a rest interval – a client who has a reading below 92 per cent saturation will need to rest until oxygen saturation increases. Monitor RPE, and advise your client to rest if it exceeds 15. If the reading does not return to a minimum of 92 per cent within 2–4 minutes of rest they will need to take on oxygen. Clients who are likely to need extra oxygen will have their own supply. The issue for the instructor is to check your organisation's health and safety policy regarding having oxygen cylinders in the gym or studio. There is no risk or danger providing the oxygen cylinder is not near a naked flame or lighted cigarette.

What is chronic obstructive pulmonary disorder (COPD)?

COPD is a term used to describe a group of conditions that have in common 'airway obstruction'. The conditions are:

- **chronic bronchitis** – inflammation of the bronchial passageways, which increases sputum production and the need to cough.
- **emphysema** – destruction and loss of elasticity of the alveoli (air sacs). The airways become narrow, which makes it difficult to absorb oxygen, causing a shortness of breath.
- **chronic asthma** – inflammation of the airways in the lungs, leading the airways to contract, caused by allergy or environmental conditions. Unlike chronic bronchitis and emphysema, asthma can be reversed and responds well to medication.

COPD clients may have the following symptoms:

- shortness of breath
- coughing with more sputum (although asthmatics have a dry cough)
- weight loss (or weight gain as a result of steroid drugs such as prednisolone)
- fatigue.

Due to shortness of breath, COPD clients are likely to be inactive and therefore deconditioned. Most COPD rehabilitation is through consultant referral, although this may differ regionally. The British Lung Foundation has a list of where the nearest group might be on their website (see online resources on page 125). The pulmonary rehabilitation course is run by specialist nurses and physiotherapists – they would welcome the opportunity to work with local fitness professionals who would continue to support COPD clients with their exercise training after they have completed their rehabilitation programme.

Exercise is considered an essential component of treatment for people with COPD. The aim of the exercise programme is to improve shortness of breath and exercise capability. The research has shown that rehabilitation relieves shortness of breath and fatigue and enhances the client's sense of control over their condition and improves exercise tolerance. Clients with COPD are likely to be highly sedentary and de-conditioned, so the programme will need to be progressed slowly at a low intensity level. In cases of severe COPD, patients can never work at high levels. An exercise class specifically for COPD clients is very beneficial because it provides clients with the security and comfort of knowing that those around them understand their limitations. The ideal class format is a circuit class where you can easily monitor the group and time periods of rest and activity (see figure 10.4 on page 122). The exercise programme for a COPD patient will also help them to improve their functional activity so that they can carry out their activities of daily living (see page 125).

Exercise recommendations

Goal

To improve breathing, to increase exercise capacity and muscle power and restore the confidence to be active and carry out activities of daily living. An important element of the programme is social and psychological support and this client group is particularly suitable for group exercise.

Cardiovascular training

Cardiovascular exercise intensity is based on RPE of 11–15. Exercise tolerance may initially be very limited, and interval training can start with as little as two minutes of exercise alternating with two minutes of rest. This can be further reduced if necessary for individual clients, but aim for two minutes initially. An important part of the CV training is to help clients change their perception of their shortness of breath. For a COPD client, becoming breathless is perceived negatively and they consider it an illness. They need to understand that breathlessness at a certain level will help improve their exercise capacity and reduce their shortness of breath in the long term. See figures 10.1–10.3 on pages 120–121 for comfortable positions to help manage shortness of breath, tightness of the chest and wheezing.

As your client's tolerance improves, increase the ratio of exercise to rest. The warm up is particularly important for clients with COPD. The goal of the warm up is to very gradually increase the heart rate so that the lungs can slowly adjust to the increased workload. A relatively constant intensity, such as walking or upright cycling, may help prevent shortness of breath. Avoid exercise that has a variable aerobic intensity.

Strength Training

A sedentary lifestyle and poor nutrition may result in muscle wasting, so strength training will start with own body resistance and progress to bands, free weights and resistance machines. Use low intensity weights that the client can lift comfortably without holding their breath.

Avoid CV, resistance and exercises that press

the contents of the stomach up against the lungs which will inhibit breathing, for example recumbent cycling.

Special considerations

- avoid excessively cold or warm environments that may trigger shortness of breath
- on days of breathing difficulties keep to low intensity activities
- use interval training
- monitor RPE
- there are some clients that may need to supplement their oxygen during training. The decision to work with clients with advanced emphysema will depend on how confident the instructor feels and also on the policy of the organisation with regard to having oxygen cylinders on the gym floor.

Client care and education

- include relaxation time as a component in your client's fitness programme. Avoid getting clients down onto the floor – it is preferable to keep them seated in a chair
- teach clients diaphragmatic breathing as set out below
- COPD clients often take up a very fixed position across the chest and the shoulders, and become very rigid and tense as they try to cope with their shortness of breath. Figures 10.1–10.3 will help relieve shortness of breath and relax your client.

Coping with a panic attack

Difficulty breathing can lead to a feeling of panic, and the following techniques help to reduce extreme breathlessness. However, it can take some time for the breath to return to normal:

Step 1
Adopt one of the above positions which will ease the work of breathing.

Step 2
Breathing technique: pursed lip breathing or 'blowing out breath'

- gently blow out – the in breath will automatically be larger
- repeat this process and breathing will return to normal.

Step 3
Diaphragmatic breathing or abdominal breathing – a relaxed breathing technique that will help slow down the breathing rate. The breaths should be natural rhythm breathing and not deep. Be aware that not all COPD clients will be able to do this exercise because their diaphragm may be too rigid as a result of their condition:

- rest hands on abdomen
- gently breathe in through the nose, and the hand on the abdomen should rise
- breathe or sigh the air out through the mouth and the hand on the abdomen should fall
- repeat these three steps while thinking about relaxing the shoulders.

NB: If a panic attack persists seek medical advice.

Figure 10.1 Breathing technique 1

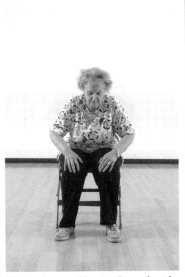

Sitting down and leaning forwards with elbows resting on thighs.

Figure 10.2 Breathing technique 2

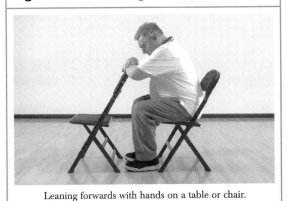

Leaning forwards with hands on a table or chair.

Figure 10.3 Breathing technique 3

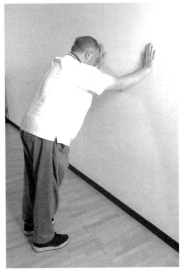

Standing and leaning against a wall.

Adaptations and modifications

Whether you are working with COPD clients in a group situation or one to one, it will help you to have an understanding of how COPD affects daily living, the physical deterioration that can occur and the psychological impact that COPD can have on a client.

Prior to rehabilitation, the COPD clients will have experienced a cycle of decline that begins with the inability to be able to breathe properly, and with that comes the fear of not being able to breathe at all. COPD sufferers often become very anxious and afraid to do any activity as it only intensifies their breathlessness. Therefore, a COPD sufferer is likely to become very sedentary and do the absolute minimum to avoid aggravating their symptoms. This can affect their ability to be able to shop, cook and generally take care of themselves, which can lead to malnutrition, muscle wasting and weakness, which results in a life overshadowed by fear, chronic anxiety and feelings of despair.

As a fitness instructor you are unlikely to be dealing with a COPD patient in the early stages of their rehabilitation unless you partner with a local pulmonary rehabilitation group. However, understanding the background and the ravaging

Figure 10.4 COPD Circuit

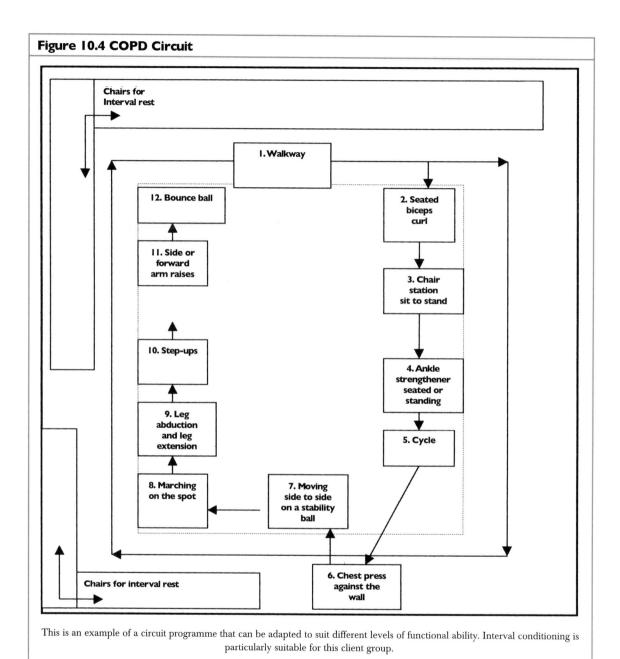

This is an example of a circuit programme that can be adapted to suit different levels of functional ability. Interval conditioning is particularly suitable for this client group.

effect of COPD on quality of life emphasises the vital role you can have in restoring a sense of worth to the life of a COPD client. Working with COPD clients can be very rewarding as you see how they progress and adapt to their condition, adjust to their perceptions of breathing limitations and go on to get the best out of life.

1. Start with gentle mobilisation and stretch, gradually enlarging movement and increasing heart rate very slowly to prepare lungs for extra workload. Monitor intensity using Rate of Perceived Exertion.
2. Start the circuit at two minutes per station followed by a two minute rest.
3. Advise clients to rest when needed.
4. Provide clients with a record sheet to write down their RPE score after each station during the rest time. Over a period of a few week this will be a useful measure of how clients are adapting, giving them a sense of achievement and it will also guide you on how you progress the intensity time or type of exercise. (See Table 10.1 for suggested options.)
5. Repeat Circuit 2-3 times.
6. Cool down with a seated relaxation and diaphragmatic breathing exercise (see the box on p. 121).

*Ankle Strengthener – Standing or seated

- Stand tall with good posture, near a wall or back of chair for support with legs three inches apart. *If seated sit tall with ribs lifted and back long.*
- Bend knees and centre weight evenly between legs. *If seated, legs are feet hip width apart with knees over ankles.*
- Transfer weight to one leg, bending the knee slightly to support the leg.
- Place the heel of your other foot on the floor then lift it and place the toes on the floor, in a heel toe action. If seated, try to increase the range of movement by aiming to put toes directly under the knees.
- Stand tall and walk on the spot and circle the ankles left then right to relieve tension.
- Repeat on the other side.

Technique
✓ Avoid banging the heel down.
✓ Gradually increase the range of movement at the joint.
✓ Try to place the toe on the exact spot where the heel was.

Table 10.1 Circuit summary for COPD	
Circuit Station	*Options*
1. Walkway	• Carry hand weights
2. Seated bicep curl	• Increase weights • Standing bicep curl
3. Sit to stand	• Lower level of seat e.g. use a stool or a step
4. Seated ankle strengthener	• Standing ankle strengthener
5. Upright cycle	
6. Chest press against the wall	• Decrease intensity by standing closer to the wall. • Increase intensity by standing further away from the wall • Increase intensity by using the edge of a steady table
7. Moving side to side on a stability ball	• Sit on stability ball • Alternate raising one arm up and opposite foot off the floor.
8. Marching on the spot	• Increase lift in knee • Hold hand weights
9. Alternating leg abduction and leg extension	• Hold on to a chair or wall for support
10. Step ups	• Carry hand weights
11. Alternating side and forward arm raises	• Without weights • With weights
12. Bounce ball seated	• Leaning forwards with elbows resting on thighs • Sitting upright • Against a wall gradually lifting arms higher

Summary

- COPD includes chronic bronchitis, emphysema, and chronic asthma
- an obstruction of the airway causes a shortness of breath that will deter people who have a condition from being active
- exercise can improve shortness of breath and increase a client's confidence to be more physically active
- interval training will provide periods of rest that can be gradually increased as exercise capability improves
- shortness of breath can be managed more easily by taking up certain positions.

Table 10.2	Exercise Summary for COPD			
Condition/mode	Cardiovascular training	Strength training	Flexibility	Additional advice
COPD	Walking, swimming, cycling, circuits. Diaphragmatic breathing.	Free weights Circuits.	Passive and active stretching, Tai Chi, Yoga.	Longer and gradual warm up and cool down allowing the lungs to adapt to changes in oxygen requirements.
Intensity/duration	RPE 11–13, 1–2 sessions 3–7 times a week; 30 minutes per session. Monitor shortness of breath.	Low resistance and high reps 2–3 days a week.	3–7 weekly.	Build up total training session to 1 hour continuous training, with shorter intervals of 5–10 minutes training with rests if required.
Goal	Improve depth of breathing and exercise tolerance.	Improve muscle strength and increase stamina for CV exercise.	Improve gait, balance and ROM. Improve depth of breathing.	Provide social opportunities and encourage interaction for social and emotional wellbeing and peer support.

Online resources

British Lung Foundation
www.lunguk.org

CORONARY HEART DISEASE (CHD)

11

It is most likely that you will come into contact with CHD clients during phase four of their rehabilitation (phases of cardiac rehabilitation set out below). With an understanding of your client's experience with this condition you will be more confident about creating an exercise programme that will maintain or improve their fitness and, of equal importance, you will keep them motivated to exercise regularly. Initially CHD clients need special care from a Cardiac Rehabilitation Nurse, who may work in conjunction with an instructor who is on the Register of Exercise Professionals (REP) and hold a British Association of Cardiac Rehabilitation (BACR) or S/NVQ Level 3 Instructor qualification.

What is coronary heart disease?

Coronary heart disease (CHD) is a condition in which the heart muscle receives inadequate blood supply. This is caused by the narrowing of the coronary arteries (referred to as coronary artery disease (CAD)). The narrowing of the arteries is a result of *atherosclerosis*, in which fatty deposits are deposited on the arterial walls and decrease the size of the arteries. This reduces blood flow and eventually the artery will become blocked and lead to an irregular heart rhythm or heart failure. Other common terms associated with CHD are:

- **myocardial infarction** (MI) is more commonly known as a heart attack, caused by interrupted blood flow to the heart and permanent muscular damage.
- **angina** is caused by reduced circulation of blood to the heart that may or may not

involve heart or artery disease. The symptoms are pain or discomfort during exertion most commonly in the chest, but could be in the jaw or arm or back. If the pain is experienced at rest or at unpredictable times exercise is not advised and refer to GP.
- **peripheral arterial disease** (narrowing of the blood vessels in the lower extremities) is caused by a reduction in blood flow to the legs and feet, making any activity painful. Exercise should not be performed unless advised by a GP or medical professional.
- **arrhythmias** changes in the rhythm of the heartbeat.

Heart attack symptoms include severe prolonged chest pain pressure that may radiate to the arms, back or neck. Other signs are sweating, nausea or vomiting.

Exercise recommendations

Goal

To build up confidence of your client to be physically active and reduce risk of secondary CHD. To provide guidance on healthy lifestyle choices with regard to diet and activity levels. To recommend exercise at least three times a week on alternate days of 20–40 minutes of interval training (see section page 38) or accumulated activity. Gradually extend periods of CV conditioning and reduce the length of active rest. After completing phase 4 of rehabilitation, clients should be able to manage continuous CV training followed by resistance training.

Instructors who are providing programmes for adults with diagnosed CHD should have the appropriate S/NVQ Level 3 or BACR qualification.

Cardiovascular training

Clients who have had a heart attack will have a lower aerobic training threshold of 50–70 per cent of their maximum heart rate. Exercise should include aerobic training of low to moderate intensity and long duration, with repetitive movement of large muscle groups, for example cycling, walking, jogging, rowing and circuit training. Medication for CHD reduces the heart rate, so use Borg's RPE scale at a maximum of 11–15 as an intensity guide. The programme content should include a 15 minute warm up, an aerobic conditioning phase of 20–30 minutes that may include resistance training if appropriate, a 10 minute cool down and a 5–10 minute relaxation session. Interval training including active rest, for example 20–40 minutes of either accumulated or continuous exercise in a group, is really suitable for these clients as it both improves physical fitness and provides an opportunity to gain social and psychological support from peers.

Strength training

Clients with stable cardiac conditions and blood pressure will benefit from low to moderate intensity resistance exercise, and it will reduce the demand on the heart during activities of daily living such as lifting and carrying, and can also be effective in improving cardiovascular health, body composition and strength. Begin with single sets of 10–15 reps 2–3 times a week and gradually build to three sets of 8–10 exercises.

Flexibility and range of movement

Range of movement and static stretches are recommended for all muscle groups. It is important to give CHD clients a 10 minute cool down before you get them lying down on the floor for stretching. Avoid any sudden movements to prevent sudden increases in blood pressure and to avoid *orthostatic hypotension* (see table 11.1 on page 128 for more details).

Orthostatic hypotension is associated with medication, and refers to the ability to regulate blood pressure in movement, which diminishes with age. Any sudden changes in movement can lead to light-headedness, dizziness and increased risk of falling.

Special considerations and screening guidelines

- monitor for abnormal signs such as chest pains, shortness of breath and dizziness
- supervision is required for moderate to high-risk patients
- clients with CHD can also have peripheral arterial disease (PAD) and diabetes. If this is the case then see the guidelines for diabetes on pages 109–13. Always seek medical advice before working with a client that has PAD.

Client care and education

- teach clients about RPE and how to monitor their intensity levels during their training session (see page 34
- advise on active rest whenever required (see interval training information on pages 38)
- reassure them that being regularly active will improve the health of their heart.

Table 11.1	The phases of cardiac rehabilitation	
	Description of phase	*What happens?*
Phase 1	Usually begins after diagnosis of an acute cardiac event such as a heart attack or heart surgery.	• medical evaluation • reassurance and education • risk factor assessment for a secondary event of heart failure.
Phase 2	Begins after discharge from hospital, during which time the patient may feel isolated, insecure and anxious.	• support provided by home visits or telephone calls from health professionals • assistance and guidance and a 'cognitive' behavioural programme • learning stress management techniques and positive lifestyle changes that will aid recovery and reduce the risk of secondary coronary heart disease.
Phase 3	Education and group exercise programmes run by a physiotherapist, occupational therapist or cardiac rehabilitation nurse, and sometimes in conjunction with an S/NVQ Level 3 or BACR qualified instructor. Local resources vary considerably and rehab programmes can range between 1 x weekly for 4 weeks to 2–3 weekly for 8–12 weeks.	• exercise includes aerobic training of low to moderate intensity and long duration with repetitive movement of large muscle groups, e.g. cycling, walking, jogging, rowing or circuit training. • sessions advised to have a 15 minute warm up, an aerobic conditioning phase of 20–30 minutes that may include resistance training if appropriate, a 10 minute cool down and a 5–10 minute relaxation session.
Phase 4	Long-term maintenance of physical exercise and lifestyle change with an S/NVQ Level 3 or BACR qualified instructor.	• GP or medical professional referral to a qualified instructor if desired by client • a continuation of phase 3 with ongoing education and exercise programming that will motivate the client to maintain regular exercise.

For more information visit www.sign.ac.uk/guidelines

Case study

Cardiac Rehabilitation – Alan's experience

I had my heart attack in early February 2004 – not a TV style clutch at chest, foam at the mouth and fall over backwards affair, but something more like heartburn which lasted for three days before I decided that an ambulance might be a good idea. Recovering in the Coronary Care Unit of Harlow's Princess Alexandra Hospital, I was introduced to the Cardiac Rehabilitation Unit – a trio of extremely enthusiastic, helpful and thoroughly professional nursing staff dedicated to getting patients of coronary heart disease back into mainstream life. It was here that I learnt about the contributing factors which amounted to:

- a significant genetic contribution (Dad died at 54 following a heart attack)
- 45 years of smoking (40 cigarettes a day just prior to the heart attack)
- high blood pressure
- a previously high stress work environment
- a very sedentary lifestyle in the three years since retirement
- little consideration to diet.

Although there was little I could do about the first factor, it was suggested that my life expectancy could be considerably extended and my general quality of life improved were I to pay some attention to the other five. It was explained that my local sports centre ran a phase III cardiac rehabilitation course, combining basic lectures on cardiology-related topics alongside circuit-based exercises designed to improve general and cardiac fitness. It would also give me the opportunity to interact with people of similar experience – people who would understand. I was enrolled!

As phase III of my cardiac rehabilitation progressed I found that I thoroughly enjoyed the exercise sessions, and that I gained a great deal from them. I had decided from the outset that if a lifestyle change was to come about, then it would be total. So out went fags and fat (the former with masses of support from the cardio team and my GP clinic) and in came exercise for two 30 minute sessions a week. Not only did a general improvement in my fitness become apparent, but my confidence was gaining strength too. As well as the realisation that I could put my body under pressure without undue ill effect, reassuring conversations with my peers on the course showed that I was not the only one suffering side effects as a result of some of the drugs that I was prescribed. I also learned where I could buy the recommended foods (oat bread for example) and how to prepare them to provide meals which are both healthy and tasty. Another invaluable lesson was that, should I ever need it, there is simply masses of support available. I was quite sorry when the course ended, but was cheered to learn that I could apply to join the phase IV group – which was supposed to be much of the same in terms of exercise, but a little more challenging.

They weren't joking! At first I found the 20 minutes warm up, 20 minutes exercise (at your own pace) and 20 minutes cool down 'challenging' to a high degree, and I really looked forward to tea afterwards and the chance to chat and compare experiences. As I became accustomed to the faster pace of phase IV (and, of course, this was the pace which I had chosen), I began to enjoy the physical exercise increasingly, to the extent that I joined the gym as a full-time member, so that I could benefit further from the equipment and coaching from the qualified instructors.

So, where am I today, 18 months after the heart attack and 12 months after starting phase IV? For starters my lifestyle has undertaken a complete U-turn! I have not smoked a cigarette in over a year, and my diet is as controlled as I want it to be (as are my blood pressure and cholesterol levels). My confidence is growing steadily – I occasionally have mini panic attacks, but since I know what they are all about I am steadily gaining control and can shrug them off relatively easily. Then, of course, there is exercise. In addition to the phase IV class, which I hate to miss for any reason, I attend the gym four times each week for a 90 minute session each time. Without exaggeration I am physically fitter than at any time in the last 20 years and am more mentally alert than I have been since I retired. I still attend the occasional outpatient clinic at Princess Alexandra Hospital where my cardiologist has said that, to all intents and purposes, my recovery is 100 per cent complete. Finally there is the support which I continue to enjoy at home, within the health service and, of course, from the group at phase IV and the staff at the sports centre.

Table 11.2	Exercise summary for CHD			
Condition/mode	Cardiovascular training	Strength training	Flexibility and range of movement	Additional advice
CHD	Cycling, walking, jogging, rowing, circuit training and interval training.	Strength training (with stable cardiac conditions and blood pressure) 3 × weekly with 48 hours rest between sessions.	ROM and static stretches – hold stretches for 20–30 seconds.	15 minute warm up, 10 minute cool down and 5–10 minute relaxation session.
Intensity/duration	Low to moderate intensity at 50–70 per cent of HR max heart or RPE 11–15. 3–7 days a week for 30–60 minutes per session.	1 set of 10–15 reps, building to 3 sets of 8–10 reps.	2–3 days a week, or before and after each training session.	Monitor for chest pains and feelings of pressure or dizziness. Supervision is required for moderate to high-risk patients. Clients with CHD are likely to have peripheral arterial disease (PAD*) or diabetes mellitus.
Goal	Increased aerobic capacity, decreased BP and HR. Decrease in CHD risk factors.	Increased muscle strength and endurance. Reduced oxygen demands of muscular activities during activities of daily living.	Improved range of motion, increased flexibility and reduced risk of injury.	Support your client psychologically by listening to how they feel. This will increase their confidence in you, which will motivate them to exercise and maintain regular activity that will reduce the risk of secondary CHD.

- Peripheral artery disease is a narrowing of blood vessels in the lower extremities, and causes pain in legs and feet. Exercise should not be performed unless advised by a GP or medical professional.

HYPERTENSION

12

Hypertension is more commonly known as high blood pressure, and is the pressure of the blood in the arteries. High blood pressure develops if the walls of the larger arteries lose their natural elasticity and become rigid and the smaller blood vessels become narrower (constrict).

In the majority of people there is no definite cause of high blood pressure. This is known as 'essential hypertension'. The following factors can also contribute to high blood pressure:

• sedentary lifestyle
• overweight
• too much salt in the diet
• drinking too much alcohol
• poor nutrition and not enough fruit and vegetables.

Blood pressure increases with age – as people age the arterial walls stiffen and have a reduced ability to constrict and dilate. The pressure against an increasingly inflexible artery wall builds up and increases the load on the heart. High blood pressure is a major risk factor for cardiovascular disease in older adults.

What is hypertension?

Blood pressure measures *systolic* and *diastolic* pressure. The heart is a pump that beats by contracting and relaxing. The pressure of blood flow through the arteries changes at different stages of the heartbeat.

• **systolic pressure** indicates pressure in the arteries when the heartbeat is forcing blood through them.
• **diastolic pressure** indicates pressure in the arteries when the heart relaxes.

There is no universal agreement as to the upper limits for normal systolic and diastolic blood pressure, especially with older adults because blood pressure increases with age (particularly systolic pressure). In western society, a resting systolic blood pressure of 160mmHg and a resting diastolic blood pressure of 90mmHg is regarded as hpertensive. However, recent guidelines (Wood *et al.*, 1998) recommend the treatment goals in the box below, as set by the British Hypertension Society.

> ### British Hypertension Society guidelines
>
> • provide advice on lifestyle modifications for all people with high blood pressure
> • drug therapy is initiated for people with a *sustained* systolic BP of 160 mmHg, or *sustained* diastolic BP of 100mmHg
> • treatment decisions are made for people with systolic BP between 140–150 mmHg and diastolic BP between 90–99mmHg
> • the goal is to maintain systolic BP <140mmHg and a diastolic BP of < 90mmHg
> • the goal for diabetics is to maintain systolic BP < 130mmHg and diastolic BP < 85 mmHg

Exercise recommendations

NB: An exercise programme for a client with high blood pressure must only commence after medication therapy has started, or on the advice of their GP.

Goals

To encourage weight loss by increasing aerobic activity to 30–45 minutes on most days of the week. To provide guidance on healthy lifestyle choices with regard to diet and saturated fat intake, smoking cessation and alcohol consumption.

Cardiovascular training

Regular low to moderate intensity aerobic endurance can reduce systolic and diastolic blood pressure. Studies have identified that training at lower intensities, i.e. 40–50 per cent of HR max, lowers blood pressure as much as training at higher intensities (Gordon, 1997). Lower intensity exercise is both safer for older adults, particularly if they have other chronic conditions, and has been shown to be as effective, if not more so, in reducing blood pressure than higher intensity exercise. Always include an extended cool down to avoid complications such as arrhythmias, angina or post exercise hypotension (see details on page 133). Be aware that medication for high blood pressure reduces heart rate, and intensity should be guided by Borg's RPE scale at a maximum of 11–15.

Strength Training

Research findings for strength training are less conclusive with regards to whether it reduces blood pressure, although it has been identified that low to moderate intensity strength training can reduce resting blood pressure, and that it may also be effective in reducing the oxygen demands of muscular activity. However, the following factors should be considered:

- avoid isometric exercises (muscular contractions against a load which is fixed or immovable), as they can increase blood pressure and heart rate to levels that would be dangerous for anyone with hypertension
- flexibility training, such as passive and active stretching, or Tai Chi, to stretch all major muscle groups is recommended three times a week.

Special considerations

- The British Association of Cardiac Rehabilitation recommends that participants should not exercise if resting systolic BP is greater than 180 mmHg or diastolic is greater than 100 mmHg and has a resting heart rate of 100bpm-plus.
- beta blockers for high blood pressure reduce the heart rate by up to 30 beats per minute and may cause *post exercise hypotension* (see table 12.2 on page 133)
- high blood pressure increases the risk of stroke
- high blood pressure is a risk factor for heart attack, stroke, heart and kidney failure and dementia
- there are several factors that can raise blood pressure temporarily, such as exercise, alcohol, caffeine, smoking, a full bladder, anxiety, excitement and pain.

Client care and education

- teach clients to monitor their RPE during their training session
- advise active rest whenever required (see interval training details on page 38)
- reassure your client that being regularly active will help keep their BP at a safe level.

Contraindications for exercise

Your client should not undertake exercise if any of the following apply:

- unstable angina
- BP > 200/100
- drop in BP during activity
- unstable heart condition
- unstable diabetes
- high temperature

Table 12.1	Common drugs used to treat cardiovascular diseases, and their effects on exercise.
ACE inhibitors (Angiotensin-converting enzyme)	ACE inhibitors work by making the walls of the arteries relax and dilate. They are most effective when used with a diuretic. They reduce the load on the heart by causing vasodilatation of the arteries (opening up the arteries) which reduces blood pressure. They can cause a drop in blood pressure (postural hypertension) on standing.
Beta blockers and calcium channel blockers	Treat cardiovascular disease including angina and hypertension. Beta-blockers and some calcium channel blockers decrease heart rate and therefore heart rate measures are not a good indicator of intensity. Rate of perceived exertion (RPE) is a more reliable way to monitor intensity of exercise. They cause tiredness and low blood pressure.
Diuretics	Diuretics are prescribed for different reasons. Some decrease blood pressure by increasing urine output, and there is an increased need to make frequent visits to the toilet. Be aware that your client may be tempted to drink less water to avoid the inconvenience and interruption during their exercise programme. Explain that exercise causes a loss of fluid through perspiration and if they don't drink water that are likely to become dehydrated. Some diuretics are prescribed for the treatment of heart conditions.
Nitrates	Dilate arteries and veins, which reduces the pressure of blood flow returning to the heart. Also dilate the arteries which reduces the after-load of the heart, but most importantly they dilate the coronary arteries, improving blood flow to the heart. Spray on medication should be taken to a training session or class for use in the event of chest pain during exercise, as nitrates can cause a sudden drop in blood pressure.

Drugs used to treat cardiovascular disease

It is very important to be aware of the effects of medications for hypertension and how they may affect your client's response to exercise. Medications for hypertension include beta-blockers, calcium channel blockers and diuretics. Establish whether your client is taking medication, and if they are experiencing any side effects such as light-headedness or sluggishness. Some medications for high blood pressure can increase the risk of *post exercise hypotension* – this may mean that a drop in blood pressure after exercise, or any sudden movements or changes in position such as standing up, may cause light-headedness. This can be avoided by extending the cooling down period of their programme, and slowly returning their heart rate and blood pressure to resting levels.

Summary

- clients with a history of cardiovascular disease have a reduced aerobic capacity
- low to moderate intensity interval training alternating aerobic training with active rest is recommended
- active rest can include resistance training, using own body resistance, hand weights, body bars and walking
- aerobic intervals should gradually increase and active rest should gradually reduce until 30 minutes of continuous exercise is achieved
- medication for cardiovascular conditions can cause *orthostatic hypotension*, causing light-headedness and dizziness, which can increase the risk of falls
- any sudden changes in movement should be avoided, and transitions between the floor and standing should be gradual
- the warm up and cool down should be extended to allow the heart rate to adjust very gradually.

Table 12.2	Exercise summary for hypertension Condition/Mode			
Condition/mode	Cardiovascular training	Strength training	Flexibility and range of movement	Additional advice
Hypertension	Walking, swimming, treadmill, circuits, upright or recumbent cycle, stair climber.	Circuits, light weights, own body resistance.	Passive and active stretching, Tai Chi.	Be aware of the effects of medication on heart rate readings.
Intensity/duration	40–80 per cent maximum heart rate (lower intensities, i.e. 50 per cent max are most effective for stabilising BP), RPE 11–15 3–7 days a week for 30–60 minutes per session.	High reps low resistance on alternate days.	3–7 days.	Extended and gradual cool down returning to resting heart rate. 15 minute warm up, 10 minute cool down and 5–10 minute relaxation session.
Goal	Lower blood pressure and increase energy expenditure. Increase speed and duration of CV exercise.	Increase or maintain strength.	Improve ROM and flexibility	

Summary of chronic conditions

- older adults are the fastest growing group of the population and are very much aware of how regular activity can improve their health and wellbeing
- there are ever increasing numbers of older adults seeking the advice and support of fitness professionals, and this number will only grow in the future
- regular exercise and specific and tailored exercise programming that is carefully considered and tailored to meet their specific needs will provide older clients with:
  - pain relief from their chronic condition
  - a positive mental attitude that will improve their quality of life
  - improvements in their cardiovascular fitness, strength, flexibility and mobility that can prevent the spiral of decline into disability
  - autonomy and independence.

Further reading

Durstine, L. J. and Moore, G. E. (2003) *ACSM's Exercise Management for Persons with Chronic Diseases and Disabilities* (Human Kinetics)

Durstine, L. J. (2002) *ACSM's Exercise Management for Persons with Chronic Diseases and Disabilities* (Human Kinetics)

Egger, G. and Champion, N. (1990) *The Fitness Leaders Handbook*, third edition (A&C Black)

Jessie Jones, C. and Rose, Debra J. (2005), *Physical Activity Instruction of Older Adults* (Human Kinetics)

Poggiali, T. and Peters, K. (2000) *Step in the Right Direction Manual* (Keiser Institute on Ageing)

Online resources

www.bpassoc.org.uk, the Blood Pressure
    Association
www.bhf.org.uk, the British Heart Foundation
www.bhsoc.org, the British Hypertension
    Society
www.britishlungfoundation.com, the British
    Lung Foundation
www.wrightfoundation.com, for information on
    medically led exercise referral programme
    qualifications.

INSTRUCTION AND PROGRAMMING SKILLS

PART **FOUR**

DEVELOPING INSTRUCTION SKILLS

13

Working with a specialist population such as older adults requires a willingness to learn new skills, a commitment to ongoing education and a genuine desire to support and care for older clients. It also requires an openness to provide support and guidance on all aspects of health, such as diet, nutrition, stress management and relaxation and to give direction on where to find specialist health or advice if required. It does not mean that you have to 'know it all'; it does mean that you need to have the willingness and are interested enough in your client to find out. Patience and tolerance will be required to repeat instruction frequently, and in some cases, all the time. Do not expect older clients to achieve perfect form after a few sessions – some may never achieve perfect form! Many older adults are beginners and they may have spent a lifetime of being unaware of their body and the mechanics of movement. It is important to remember that medication can sometimes affect memory recall and reaction time. Showing compassion for their difficulties will give them the confidence and motivation to keep coming back. The best part of teaching older adults is that you can genuinely and positively impact their health and lifestyle choices, making a real difference to their quality of life, and they will be very appreciative.

Advanced preparation and planning

Write a plan

Know in advance what you intend to do, either in a one to one session or in a group session. Set out your plan in sequential order and allocate time scales. This will make you think more realistically about what you want to achieve and how much time you need. Having clear goals will keep both you and your client or group focused, and make you appear professional. This does not mean that your session has to become regimented – build in time that allows for conversation and sharing a couple of jokes. Socialising and fun is an important part of psychological wellbeing and mental health.

Decide on activities

Plan your activities – the moves and music, the cardiovascular or resistance equipment – and think about how you can accommodate different fitness abilities and adapt for chronic conditions. Knowing in advance what you are going to do and having alternative options up your sleeve is a sign of a true professional, and will instil confidence in your client or group.

Prepare the equipment

Organise in advance any props that you will need, such as steps, bands, balls, hand weights, body bars and balance boards. Have them ready, or readily accessible, precisely as you need them. This will ensure your session is time efficient and transitions from your planned sequence of exercises run smoothly.

Know what you want to say

If you are teaching an exercise to music class, practise your moves in advance and identify at which phrase and count you intend to cue new moves or provide teaching points. Exceptional teachers know how to get the best out of their class and use:

- timing
- rehearsed phrases
- cueing skills
- visual and verbal cues.

Planning what to say in advance and keeping a record of teaching points and cues will provide a solid and professional basis for you to teach. You can build on the preparations and add a spontaneous and fun element that will work with the mood and energy of your class.

Use professional instruction

In a group situation it is the instructor's responsibility to make everyone feel at ease, and not the other way round. Always greet the group with an upbeat tone, a simple hello with a smile. Communicate with every single person in the room and make eye contact with each and every participant during the session. The following points can help:

- scan the group for new faces and speak to new people individually. Make yourself open to them asking questions, reassure them about what they will be doing and screen them for any injuries or conditions.
- in one to one situations ask them how they are and hear their reply. Listen to their tone of voice – is it flat or upbeat? Do they *sound* like they feel well? Look at their eyes to see how they feel – do they hold a story of pain, or are they bright eyed and raring to go? How is their posture – are they standing tall or slightly stooped? Recognise the signs of how they are feeling – show empathy, give reassurance and adapt your training session accordingly.

The following tips will allow you to communicate effectively:

- **tell the group what you are going to do and why you are going to do it.** Give your clients the reasons behind your exercise. You will know their history because you will have written it down, so where possible relate your instructions to group or individual goals, which will give your clients an added purpose to increase their effort.
- **equipment technique instruction.** Take your time with instructions of how to use equipment, and build up information gradually. Demonstrate what you want them to do and support their efforts, *but do not do it for them.* It takes patience and tolerance on the instructor's part to encourage independence by letting them set up the equipment themselves, however long it takes! Get your client to repeat the steps a couple of times and, if necessary, write down step-by-step instructions for them to follow and keep. Although CV equipment does give guidance it still can be difficult to follow for those with poor eyesight and a lack of confidence.
- **technique, instruction and form.** It will take time for some of your older clients to develop the body awareness required for certain exercises, especially using hand weights. You can assist their learning by regularly reviewing a bank of teaching points and cues that you write down. Work on clarity of instruction and be specific on how the activity or exercise should feel and look.

Kinaesthetic cues

Kinaesthetic or feeling cues will help your client understand how the exercise or movement should feel, and will heighten body awareness of a specific body part or action. Kinaesthetic cues can enhance the enjoyment of the exercise, and help the client to connect to their movements, creating more flow and ease of movement. For example:

- 'keep your knees soft'
- 'feel your feet sink into the ground'
- use soft movement descriptions such as 'move slowly, gently, softly'
- action cues such as calm the breath
- strong cues to emphasise a feeling of strength and power, for example 'feel the power and energy in your legs'.

Body position cues

Precise cues on the position of body parts, in relation to others will reduce risk of injury and improve alignment and posture. For example:

- starting position – feet hip width apart, toes pointing straight ahead and shoulders in line with hips
- lunges – front knee in line with ankle, back knee in line with hips pointing towards the floor
- bicep curl – tuck elbow into waist and lift palms towards the shoulders. Keep wrist in line with shoulder.

Alignment and form cues

- keep the chest lifted
- lengthen the spine
- draw the abdominals in

- drop the shoulders down away from the ears
- lengthen the neck
- slide the shoulder blades down the back and lengthen the neck
- create space between the shoulder blades
- lift the collar bone.

Health and safety and first aid

When working with older adults you need to be aware of the signs and symptoms that indicate that exercise should cease, and have the ability to ascertain if medical help should be called for. A first aid qualification will teach you the practical skills, and give you more confidence to enable you to deal with an emergency situation. It is important to recognise that older adults are at a higher risk of having a heart attack or an injury from falling or over-exertion. You also need to be aware of any conditions that are contraindicated for exercise, and be alert to health and safety hazards in the environment. Emergency situations are rare but they do happen. The instructor who regularly refreshes their knowledge and remains observant of their clients and the environment is in a position to respond appropriately. See Chapters 6–7 for screening guidelines and contraindications for chronic conditions.

A HOLISTIC WELLBEING APPROACH

14

The diverse needs of older adults

To be seen as approachable and accessible to older adults it is important to recognise that the older adult market spans four decades, and that the generation gap creates individuals with a different set of beliefs, values, and attitudes. Older adults are not all the same, and the way to motivate one individual to be regularly active may not be the way to motivate another. However, broad age groups have been outlined below to give a general overview of the approach you may wish to take – individual differences will need to be accounted for by the instructor.

People in the same age group do often share common ground as they will have grown up in the same political environment and have lived through the same historical events. It will improve your relationships with your older adults if you are familiar with issues and viewpoints that are shared by them. With this understanding you will be able to apply *behaviour change principles* that will promote adherence to exercise (see pages 144–52).

When screening your client and identifying goals, be sensitive to their broader life and wellbeing needs. For example, an older adult who has a very busy and full life may use their exercise to retreat into a haven of peace, preferring to exercise alone. Another client may need the social interaction and support of a peer group – especially those who are bereaved or live alone.

Mid life adults 45–60 years old

People in this age group will be more motivated by goals that will prevent the early onset of chronic conditions, or be an intervention for a condition in its early stages. Research from the Health Development Agency has identified that mid-life adults, many of whom are still at work, tend to be rather overlooked – not just by the fitness industry, but by society in general.

> 'You're in a group of the forgotten really, you know they do an awful lot for younger people and children and once you get over a certain age as a pensioner, then you get a lot more support. But I think for my age group there's not a lot going on, you know. We're sort of forgotten really'.
>
> *A 55-year-old research participant*

Adults 50–65 years old

People in this age group consider themselves a distinct generation with particular preferences and needs that are not recognised in public services. The do not identify themselves as 'older people' and generally feel ignored. As a group, they are the most susceptible and open to change, as the signs of ageing are all around them. Their personal experiences of the visible signs of ageing and the frailty of their parents ring alarm bells – ageing is real and getting older really does happen! People in their fifties are experiencing multiple changes and transitions, such as decisions about work and employment, illness and death of parents, children leaving home and becoming grandparents. The awareness of growing older means that people in this age group are receptive to improving their fitness and health, which will lead them to a more independent, healthier old age. They want the opportunity to reflect and consider their future and plan what they will need for a healthy old age. They want to take control of their own health and wellbeing and want to have a range of opportunities and services that will help them achieve this.

Older adults 65–70 years old

People in this age group are more likely to be experiencing a decline in their health and wellbeing, and may be living with one or two chronic conditions. Their goal will be to feel better and maintain a level of fitness and wellbeing that will keep them independent and mobile. Senior adults 70-plus will be focused more on functional fitness actions such as walking, climbing stairs, bending and reaching.

Your programme for older adults should not *just be about exercise*. Adults over the age of 60 need to be motivated by a much broader range of services. Providing the perfect exercise programme will not necessarily be enough for your older members. The physical health benefits of the exercise programme you provide need almost to be a side effect of a more complete approach to wellbeing that provides for the **social, educational, spiritual and emotional work/life balance** as well as physical development.

Social

The social side of your programme will provide vital social support and friendship opportunities for all your clients. You can also create social opportunities in the way you design your equipment layout in the gym, for example by grouping equipment in ways that makes interaction possible. Group classes, such as circuits or exercise to music, offer opportunities to bring people together for pair work and will encourage people to talk. Encouraging outdoor group activities when the weather is good, such as racket games or country walks, can encourage socialising, and a coffee morning could provide another opportunity to establish new friendships.

Educational

Helping your older adults to increase their knowledge and understanding on a broader range of health issues, and showing a willingness to find out answers to their health questions, will encourage loyalty and commitment and keep them motivated to exercise. Regular classes specifically dedicated to educating your clients on healthy eating, back care, stress management and the health benefits of regular physical activity will keep them informed and up to date with current health information and bring them together socially.

Work/life Balance

You will have a great deal to offer clients who are still at work. Mid-life adults (aged 45–60) can feel ignored, that there is not much available to them. Many older adults are still working very hard and are not in a position to retire early. If you can provide a warm and comfortable environment that encourages relaxation, and teach breathing and relaxation techniques (see pages 157–60) you will give your older clients much appreciated space and time to relax. In addition to this, the exercise programmes and education you provide will help and support members who are keen to return to work following an operation, injury or illness.

Emotional and psychological

- for many older adults, ageing can be dominated by a feeling of loss. There are the physical losses that have been covered in chapters 1–2. There can also be a loss of friends, health, income, careers, spouse and family.
- previous habits such as poor diet, smoking and alcohol abuse can begin to have an impact and intensify the normal declines and physiological changes of ageing. There can be the added anxiety and pressure to give up a habit like smoking or drinking, which involves yet more sacrifices.
- these major life changes and losses can lead to increased depression and anxiety for older adults. Some will accept these changes as a natural process while others will become afraid, anxious and depressed.

It is also important to consider the experience of older adults who have been active and lived a healthy lifestyle all their life, but have then suffered a heart attack or stroke, or become restricted by arthritis. Not surprisingly, older adults can become disillusioned, as well as afraid of over-exerting themselves and making their condition worse (see spiral of decline on page 78). There are also older adults whose lives become transformed when they observe the warning signs of the onset of a chronic condition, work with their symptoms and use the event to start a new phase in their life. Examples of these people can be found in cardiac and COPD rehabilitation on pages 129 and 122.

Relaxation, meditation and breathing techniques can also provide the space for emotional and spiritual reflection, which will become increasingly important for many older adults. This will give your clients some much needed space and time to reflect and collect themselves, adding to their overall sense of wellbeing and may encourage them to visit you more often.

Mind and body activities such as Tai Chi and yoga (covered in pages 67–9) combine physical activity to help focus on 'being in the moment' and use breathing to calm and still the mind.

Case study

The case study outlined below refers to an individual referred to the Activity for Life programme at Harlow Sportcentre, and illustrates how educational, emotional and physical benefits of the programme combine to create total wellbeing.

A 62-year-old woman was referred by her GP with cervical spondylosis, which resulted in lower back pain. She was finding the daily tasks of living very painful, particularly the lifting that was required by her job in a coffee shop. When not working, she was sedentary, which aggravated her back problem further.

The principle aim of her exercise programme was to increase suppleness, and she was guided through the back care programme ensuring gradual mobility and strength work.

- an emphasis on correct lifting technique and posture (educational) has made her employment and overall lifestyle more enjoyable as well as pain free
- as a result, she was able to return to her childhood passion of dancing (emotional and physical benefits) thanks to her own determination and commitment to a specific exercise programme.

The total wellbeing approach on her programme enabled her to continue working, and educated her on back care techniques, allowing her to reap the emotional benefits of dancing, and increased her physical activity.

NHS research (*Taking Action – improving the health and wellbeing of people in mid life and beyond*) has shown what motivates mid life adults, the services they would like to access and approaches taken by organisations who are running successful older adult programmes in the fitness industry. Some of the major factors are:

- a welcoming atmosphere
- provision of free health checks
- staff with well developed interpersonal and communication skills such as active listening, enabling and supporting
- a range of services, educational workshop, financial advice, regular health checks and social opportunities
- outreach presentations in the workplace – tell your potential clients face to face how you can help them improve their health
- information and advice – providing health and fitness education in the workplace will give them the knowledge that will help them make decisions and take control of their health
- health partnerships with other health agencies, for example GPs, physiotherapists, cardiac rehabilitation nurses, consultants and well woman clinics

THE PRINCIPLES OF BEHAVIOUR CHANGE TO MOTIVATE OLDER ADULTS

15

It is widely accepted that regular physical activity is an important component of a healthy lifestyle, yet it can still be very difficult to motivate sedentary people to exercise on a regular basis. A growing body of research suggests that specific behavioural factors may increase motivation for exercise, and people giving up. The major factors are as follows:

Social support

Social support from family and friends has been associated with long-term exercise adherence. Peer support, buddy systems, bring a friend, tell a friend and instructor follow up are examples that help older adults overcome any barriers or fears they may have, and encourage them to re-evaluate their beliefs regarding physical activity.

Self efficacy

Self efficacy refers to the confidence that older clients have regarding their ability to participate in an exercise programme, and their belief in themselves to be able to do what is asked of them. If an older adult has self efficacy then they will be willing to participate in an exercise programme or class. The effects of ageing such as changes in appearance and the onset of medical conditions can erode self efficacy and heighten feelings of depression. They may feel that they have no control of what is happening to them and consequently there is a loss of confidence. Older adults are far more likely to begin and maintain an exercise programme if they feel confident about their ability to succeed. Help your client to feel capable and show them success, however small, as soon as possible. Provide constant feedback during the induction and book regular monitoring and feedback appointments. These do not need to be lengthy or time consuming meetings. Learn the value of five minutes – a few brief moments of focused attention on your client will not only help you identify how they are progressing and if there is a need to review their programme, it can also keep you client motivated and inspire them to keep going. Make sure your client feels safe and be sensitive to signs of anxiety and nervousness, and always be ready to reassure respectfully without patronising them.

Promoting self efficacy

- set short-term and long-term goals that are achievable – *set your client up for success*
- use encouragement and show *genuine* belief and confidence in your client – older adults do not want or need to be patronised
- introduce your client to people who, like them, were very unsure but overcame their fears and have benefited from an exercise programme.

Activity choices

Provide a variety of opportunities to participate in physical activity and build in activity choices. Find out the interests of your client, and build that into the programme. Some clients may prefer group activities while others may prefer to exercise independently, or maybe a combination of both will be more effective. Try not to limit your exercise programme to the gym; a favoured activity of many older adults is walking and any activities that may take them outside in the fresh air. For variety set up table tennis or mat bowls indoors to provide a new interest and social contact. Research has shown that choice and variety of both the activity and location improves retention.

Health contracts

Health contracts have been shown to increase a client's commitment to their exercise programme. At the initial and screening stage when you are completing the physical activity readiness questionnaire (PAR Q) (see page 69) set out clear achievable short- and long-term goals that are guided by the desires of your client. Break the goal down into stages of achievement or 'milestones' and set timescales and review dates (see *screening and goal setting* on page 149–51).

Regular feedback

Keep a record of progress and achievement, and point out to your client how far they have come on the way to reaching their goals. Provide frequent and accurate feedback that is relevant to your client's goals, focus on the positive steps they made and encourage and reinforce their long-term aims. Research has shown that clients who engage in self monitoring are more likely to change health behaviours (Boutelle, Kirschen, Baum, 1998).

Positive reinforcement

Positive reinforcement is the way in which you reward your client, and can be as simple as acknowledging and recognising their achievements. Other ways to positively reinforce clients are by offering rewards for attendance or reaching a goal and public recognition, for example their story and picture on the notice-board or in the local newspaper. Any positive reinforcement you can give will increase your client's commitment to exercise.

Barriers to exercise

- walking and gardening are cited most often by older adults as their favoured activities
- approximately two-thirds of older women and men prefer physical activities that can be undertaken outside a formal class or group setting (King, Castro et al., 2002 and Wilcox, King, Brassington & Ahn, 1999)
- it is important to have an understanding of the barriers older adults can have to face – these barriers may be psychological, environmental, exercise and activity related and health related.

Psychological barriers

Psychological barriers refer to beliefs and attitudes towards exercise, and perceptions of exercise. Some older adults will consider exercise, and being active generally, to be hard work and best avoided. Adults over the age of 65 grew up in a culture that aimed to minimise physical activity, and were the first generation to benefit from all manner of labour saving devices such as automatic washing machines and electrical garden equipment etc. They may associate physical activity with hard work, and their aim is to make it as easy as possible. If you add to this perhaps a bad experience, or previous lack of achievement in a sport or exercise related activity, it can amount to a total lack of interest and confidence in exercising.

Environmental barriers

Environmental barriers to exercise are the outside influences that affect motivation and accessibility. For example, support from friends and family, transportation, safety in the community with safe areas to go walking or cycling. Family and friends are very influential and can be either a positive or negative influence on a person's motivation and confidence to exercise. If someone close to your client feels threatened by the fact that their friend or companion is enjoying life out of their company, they may come up with all manner of horror stories about terrible pain and injury caused by too much exercise!

Activity and exercise barriers

Activity and exercise barriers to exercise underline the importance of developing 'individual programmes' tailored to the goals, interests and fitness levels of the client. If the programme causes discomfort, muscle soreness or exceeds the client's ability in any way, their experience can become the next new horror story to spread the barriers to exercise virus! Research has found that the majority of older adults prefer low to moderate activities such as walking and gardening, and two-thirds of older women prefer to be active outside a formal group. For the one-third that do prefer group exercise, the biggest motivating factor is social interaction. An exercise programme that relates to wider interests and enhances other activities for both daily living and other leisure activities such as golf or bowling is key to overcoming this barrier.

Health related barriers

Health related barriers to exercise can be reinforced by psychological factors and environmental influences. Genuine fears of injury or pain and low energy reserves can prevent adults from being active. Any slight discomfort will be cause for alarm and you will

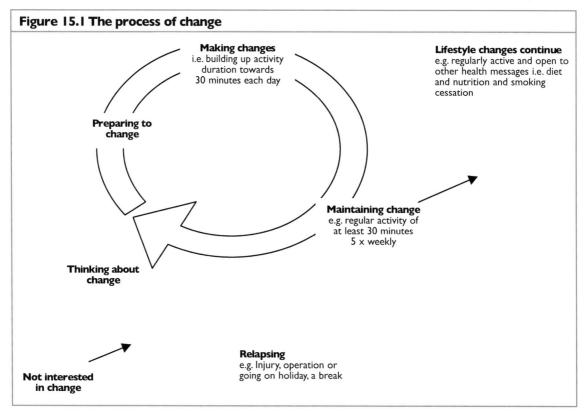

Figure 15.1 The process of change

Making changes
i.e. building up activity
duration towards
30 minutes each day

Lifestyle changes continue
e.g. regularly active and open to
other health messages i.e. diet
and nutrition and smoking
cessation

Preparing to
change

Maintaining change
e.g. regular activity of
at least 30 minutes
5 x weekly

Thinking about
change

Relapsing
e.g. Injury, operation or
going on holiday, a break

Not interested
in change

need to help your client recognise that mild aches and tension that are felt while stretching will not harm them.

Stages of change

One of the aims of a health and fitness professional is to provide the knowledge, instruction and support that will provide clients with lifestyle choices. If the client believes that it will improve their life to be more active they will make a 'behaviour change', by giving up their sedentary lifestyle and replacing it with a more active one. The 'stages of change' outlined in the Prochaska and Di Clementes's model below (1982; 1983) will help you identify exactly where a person is in the process of change. Although

your support and knowledge will do a lot to inspire and motivate your client, the process of change can be a path of many twists and turns. Your response to this process can make all the difference to a relapsed client who can be either forgotten forever, or retrieved back into the fold of active living when they are ready.

The fitness professional has a role to play in every stage of change, and can offer their support and knowledge to help a person move on. A hard sell is not required – a quiet and calm presentation of the facts that are relevant to the client will help them make their decision.

The following table gives an explanation of the process of change, and outlines actions that can be taken by the instructor to help move clients to the next stage.

Table 15.1	Action for the stages of change
Stage of change	Instructor action
Not interested in change Does not want to change current behaviour at the moment and does not plan to in the near future.	• discuss reasons and barriers to activity • feed back any information you have regarding their barriers, e.g. 'my back is too painful' could be responded to with simple and educational advice about posture and core stability in daily living • outline a programme idea that you think would help their symptoms • leave it open ended and for them to contact you if they would like some help.
Thinking about change Weighing up the pros and cons of becoming more active. When the pros start to outweigh the cons there will be a move towards preparation. The final decision to move into action can be influenced by: – **environment** – a major life event such as divorce, bereavement, or children leaving home – **new information** – a health incident such as a heart attack or a chronic condition.	• describe the benefits in relation to their specific goals • encourage them to involve their family, spouse or a friend • get a commitment to meet up and discuss their needs in more detail.

Table 15.1	Action for the stages of change cont.
Stage of change	**Instructor action**
– **priorities change –** a psychological shift in priorities, meaning that the benefits of change are perceived as important.	
Preparing to change Tries out the new behaviour – may go walking at lunch time or visit a health club to see what is on offer.	*Screening (see page 149)* • identify goals • arrange a date to introduce their programme • first session.
Making change Takes up membership or regular attendance of a class and is regularly active.	• review • provide support and identify modifications and adaptations that may be needed • setting and meeting long- and short-term health and fitness goals.
Maintaining Change	• regular reviews • exploring other health behaviour choices such as diet and nutrition, smoking cessation etc.
Relapsing Relapse is probably the most common complaint of the fitness industry – it often occurs and it is part of the process of change. There are lessons to be learned from a relapse, and we can identify times or factors that cause a relapse. High risk situations for a relapse are: – an injury – an operation – lack of support – bad weather – family demands – going on holiday.	Sometimes life situations make physical activity impossible or life circumstances make getting to a class or session difficult. Such times can be prepared for with coping strategies already in place. For example, if family obligations make it difficult to attend a class, a temporary home programme of activity can be devised with the instructor and the occasional supportive phone call will help your client remain motivated. Such commitment to your client's wellbeing will reap rewards, *especially with older clients.*

Screening and goal setting for older adults

The screening stage is the foundation of the relationship, and you can learn a great deal about your client's needs, fears and motivations by asking the right questions and using good observational skills. It is important that the screening procedure is unhurried and allows time for the older clients to become relaxed and at ease. It is important to get to know your client, to find out how they are feeling, what is motivating them and if they have any concerns about exercising. A sensitive fitness professional who is genuinely interested will make a difference to the motivation of an older adult to exercise.

Find out the following information using a relaxed and informal approach. Try to be conversational, and avoid a 'tick off the checklist' tone of voice that is used when going through the screening for health conditions. You want to get to know your client and anything about them that will help you write an exercise programme for them.

Table 15.2	Older adult motivations for exercise
Health reasons that motivate older adults to exercise: • to improve overall health • to reduce risk of disease rehabilitation • to maintain or improve mobility • to lose or maintain weight • to reduce the risk of falls.	
Psychological reasons that motivate older adults to exercise: • to feel good physically • to relieve depression • to maintain social contact and social support • to enjoy the challenge • to enjoy being active.	
Daily living activities that motivate older adults to exercise: • to maintain or improve daily living activities • to improve and maintain strength • to have more energy • to live life fully • to improve appearance.	

Table 15.3	Getting to know your client
1. What is their attitude to physical activity?	• Do they take part in any physical activity or exercise? • Do they enjoy it? • Is there an activity they particularly enjoy or enjoyed in the past? Are there any anxieties about exercising?
2. Is there any physical activity they do each day?	This is where you can talk about how valuable daily living activities are for 'accumulate fitness', and that even short periods of activity can add up and are as important to keeping fit as an exercise programme: 3 x 10 minutes or 2 x 15 minutes of housework or gardening. This approach is useful for very sedentary adults and those who have a fear of exercise
3. Identify your client's personal objectives	• Does the activity have any other leisure activities that can be enhanced by specific exercise? • How does your client cope with daily living activities such as shopping, housework, or walking up and down stairs? The aim is to relate the programme to the tasks they want to do.
4. Set SMART health and fitness goals	• SMART goals are specific, measurable, achievable, and realistic and time lined (see page 151 for more details).
5. Set behavioural goals	• Behavioural goals are those that involve commitment to action. They include time planning around class times and sessions that are put in the diary. They are times when physical activity is the priority and are scheduled into a busy routine.
6. Create a health contract and identify any situations that may cause a relapse.	Health contracts are a two-way commitment that reflects mutual respect in the client/instructor relationship: • the instructor will commit to helping the client achieve agreed goals, will support and advise and regularly review progress and will help the client overcome any barriers they may come up against • the client commits to attending their class or sessions, and any other agreed activity that can be accumulated in daily living activities. The client will let the instructor know of any unforeseen circumstances or otherwise that will prevent attendance, so that an alternative plan can be put in place – such as a home-based activity programme and telephone support.
7. Self monitoring	Research has shown that clients who monitor themselves are more likely to change health behaviours. Provide your client with a means to record their RPE against the activity, and write down how they felt.
8. Follow up	The three Cs: regular Contact, genuine Care and Consistency of the instructor will increase adherence to exercise.

Goal setting

Setting targets and goals that can be measured and evaluated are key for maintenance of behaviour change and long-term adherence to an active lifestyle. It is important that the goals come from the client; the instructor can help by asking questions that encourage the client to think about what daily living activities are affected by inactivity or a chronic condition. The client can be led towards identifying goals that will improve their activities of daily living or other leisure activities. Long-term goals such as weight loss can take a long time. Break down the goal into short-term goals or milestones that can be achieved in relatively shorter times, and play up all the other benefits of the activity that the client has experienced for themselves, for example feeling better and having more energy. Goals need to be specific to the client's needs and daily living activities. Table 15.4 shows how an initial and rather vague goal of 'wanting to feel better' turned into four very clear goals that can be measured:

1. waking up without aches and pains
2. bowling would be easier
3. join a rambling club
4. a feeling of achievement

All of the above goals could be progressed towards within the safety of a gym environment, and alongside a knowledgeable instructor, and must contain the following factors:

- **measurable** – so that the benefits and achievements are clearly visible to the client, and to know if the goals are met. Self-monitoring through record keeping and writing down feelings and RPE can also improve motivation and adherence.
- **achievable** – the exercise programme must be within the client's capabilities and be achievable within the time frame the client has available.
- **realistic** – the goals need to be based on the reality of the client's life. They can be very enthusiastic at the outset, and then other life demands creep in and the exercise programme is the first thing to be dropped. The other consideration is that over-enthusiasm can lead to over-exertion, which can result in injury and a relapse into a sedentary lifestyle.

The following table is an example of how clients can be encouraged to be more specific so that goals can become measurable, achievable and realistic.

Table 15.4	Goal setting
Specific	*Setting the goals:* **Instructor:** What would you like to get from the programme that I will design for you? **Client:** To feel better and healthier **Instructor:** So what do you feel would make you feel better and healthier? **Client:** I would like to be able to walk further **Instructor:** And how would walking further make you feel better? **Client:** I would have a feeling of achievement and of feeling well. **Instructor:** Is there anything else you would like to feel better about? **Client:** Waking up without aches and pains, and a sense that I can do what I want to do [self efficacy]. **Instructor:** Is there anything specific that you want to do? **Client:** Bowling would be easier – I could play more often – and I would be interested in joining a rambling club if I knew that I could keep up.
Behavioural and short term goals set the client up for success	• I will walk 2,000 steps every other day after breakfast • I will stretch and do mobility exercise before and after my steps • I will record my RPE when I walk, stretch and do my mobility exercises • I will write down how I feel.
Long term goals	A strength, flexibility and mobility training programme, including some balance training, will improve fitness and agility for *bowling* and a gradual increase in steps will improve *self efficacy* to join a *rambling club*. A general increase in activity will lead to an improved sense of wellbeing and perception of aches and pains.
Measurable	• use a pedometer to measure steps • self monitoring RPE and encouraging them to record their number of steps and how they feel will heighten their awareness of what they are achieving.
Achievable	The steps set, the time (after breakfast) and record keeping are agreed and within the capabilities of the client.
Realistic	Be aware that over-enthusiasm can promote unrealistic goal setting, which will have to be managed. For example, the above client may feel they can achieve 5,000 steps. The advice would be to start off gently and increase the steps by 500 a day if they feel able, but they should first see how they respond to the activity.

THE HEART AND SOUL OF
PROGRAMMING FOR OLDER ADULTS 16

This guide has given you options to dip into and select the information you are interested in, and what you need to know. There are statistics, theories, science, principles of training, psychology, an insight into chronic conditions and practical instruction advice and direction for further training.

You will make a real difference when working with older adults. It will add a depth to your teaching, and can prove to be exceptionally rewarding.

What follows is breathing techniques that help people to feel calmer and scripts for relaxation. The breathing exercises and scripts for relaxation are tried, tested and always a favourite with older clients. They provide time to be still, calm and peaceful.

Relaxation

Introducing formalised relaxation techniques to an exercise programme or group class is the final piece of the fitness jigsaw. By doing so, you give permission to your client to relax. Many people feel unable to relax, and can feel guilty if they take time out for themselves. Relaxation is another component of fitness that allows the mind and body to completely rest and, if included regularly in a busy lifestyle, it will improve mental wellbeing, relieve stress and can help to soothe and manage chronic pain.

Relaxation and meditation can be quite appealing to older adults, who are often in a more reflective phase of their lives and may need some time to turn inwards to find peace and fulfilment. Self knowledge can be gained

with regular relaxation and meditation, and the use of breathing helps the mind to be still and relaxed.

The benefits of relaxation for older adults

- recharges the batteries after physical activity
- helps the mind keep events and thoughts in perspective
- helps promote emotional and physical healing
- increases feeling of personal control
- helps relieve stress before taking it out on others
- builds resilience to stress
- puts more energy into leisure time
- improves quality of sleep
- silences thinking
- soothes and relieves pain
- helps pain management.

Relaxation and heart rate exercise

The following exercise will really bring home to your client or class participants the value of taking time out to relax. Try it out for yourself before you teach it. Clients really do enjoy this one

1. time the group or client while they count how many breaths they have in one minute (one breath includes inhalation and exhalation)
2. either write down or ask the client to remember how many breaths completed
3. go through one of the following relaxation techniques, and then ask the clients to recount their breath.

4. you will find that the majority of people will have a significantly decreased heart rate.

Three approaches to relaxation

Jacobson's progressive muscle relaxation (PMR)

PMR was developed by Dr Eric Jacobson for patients that were unable to release tension. The technique is to contract and then release each muscle group. This method can teach people the difference between tension and relaxation and is excellent for development of body and muscle awareness. It can also be used during everyday activities to release muscle tension.

Autogenic relaxation technique (ART)

ART was devised by a psychiatrist, J.H. Schultz, and uses a number of simple exercises that help to 'switch off tension' and 'switch on relaxation'. Autogenics places importance on belief in your own inner voice and innate capacity.

Meditative relaxation method

The aim of meditation is to achieve a quietening of the mind, and a heightened awareness. Regular meditation can bring greater control over restless thoughts and emotions and improve wellbeing. Simple meditation involves breathing control, and focusing the attention on either a word or an object.

Using your voice for relaxation

For relaxation to be successful, the instructor has to be authentic and speak in their natural tone. If you are genuine in your wish to help your clients to relax, that will be conveyed through your voice. You will naturally adopt a

quieter tone and a slower pace as you sense the quietening of the group. The main point is to take your time, slow your own pace down and listen to the atmosphere, which will tell you when to pause, and when to speak. The most important thing is to 'be yourself'. Helping a group to genuinely relax is very fulfilling and for many of your clients it will be the highlight of their session.

Relaxation scripts for use with your clients can been found in appendix one on pages 157–60.

Breathing techniques

The following breathing techniques can either be introduced into a relaxation class and be followed by one of the relaxation scripts (see pages 157–60), or they can be given to clients to do at the end of their session in the gym or class.

NB: *for clients with breathing difficulties and COPD conditions use the breathing techniques on pages 120–21.*

Slow breathing
- inhale, slowly counting to see how long you breathe in for
- at the end of the inhalation, pause for half a second
- now exhale, counting slowly and quietly to yourself
- after the exhalation, stop, and feel your muscles relax
- repeat the above steps and focus on the calmer and more relaxed feeling you are experiencing.

Controlled breathing

- sit well supported, or lie comfortably – relax your abdomen
- place one hand on your navel and one hand on your upper chest (have elbows supported if possible)
- breathe out fully, and let your breath go
- breathe in very gently, taking longer than you did exhaling, and feel your belly rise underneath your hand
- breathe out again gently, taking longer than you did inhaling – feel your belly drop back down
- pause for a moment
- repeat from the beginning

This technique can be used to induce tranquillity, is calming before bedtime and can reduce discomfort or pain.

Balloon breathe or rubber man

This technique is used to relax the whole body:

- loosen clothing, and sit or lie comfortably
- breathe out fully and let your breath go
- slowly breathe in, imagining as you do that you are inflating from your toes up through your legs, up through your body to your arms and fingers, and eventually to your head and face
- hold and pause for a brief moment
- breathe out slowly, picturing yourself deflating gradually and becoming soft and heavy
- rest

APPENDIX ONE
RELAXATION SCRIPTS

SCRIPT FOR PROGRESSIVE MUSCLE RELAXATION

- give your client the option to sit or lie down
- if sitting, their head needs to be supported
- hands and arms spread comfortably alongside, and away from, the body
- the key to this method is that you build the tension slowly, and release quickly
- you can play calming music in the background if you wish.

Lie down and breathe slowly and deeply. As you breathe out feel your body soften as the tension begins to leave your body. Visualise the tension as a mist drifting away from you.

Concentrate on your feet – press them down into the floor or mat as hard as you can.

Hold – feel the tension – release.

Now concentrate on your knees – press them together as firmly as you can.

Hold – feel the tension – release.

Now concentrate on your waist – draw your waist in firmly and press your belly towards your spine.

Hold – feel the tension – release.

Now concentrate on your shoulders – press them both equally into the mat or chair.

Hold – feel the tension – release.

Now concentrate on your elbows – press them down firmly into the mat.

Hold – feel the tension – release.

Now concentrate on your hands – clench them as hard as you can.

Hold – feel the tension – release.

Now stretch your hands and fingers as long and as wide as they will go.

Hold – feel the tension – release.

Now concentrate on your head – gently push your head into the mat or chair.

Hold – feel the tension – release.

Now concentrate on your eyes – shut them tightly and screw up your face.

Hold – feel the tension – release.

Now concentrate on your eyebrows – frown hard.

Hold – feel the tension – release.

Now concentrate on your jaw – clench your teeth together.

Hold – feel the tension – release.

(Teeth should now be slightly apart).

Bring your attention to your breathing – in through the nose and out through your mouth. Breathe out as slowly as you can. Repeat one more time.

You feel very relaxed, softer and warm. Rest comfortably for a few minutes.

Become aware of the ground beneath you and the space around you. Come round slowly, gently stretching.

Slowly come up into a sitting position.

[NB: If the tensing method of progressive muscular relaxation aggravates pain in your clients, then try autogenic relaxation on the next page.]

SCRIPT FOR AUTOGENIC RELAXATION

Lie down on your back, or sit comfortably in the chair. Place your arms at your sides with palms facing upwards. Take a moment to allow your body to soften into the mat or chair.

Focus all your attention on your breathing and as you inhale and exhale silently, repeat, deeper, longer, slower, repeat.

Focus all your attention on your left shoulder and silently in your mind repeat the following:

My right shoulder is heavy and relaxed
My right shoulder is heavy and relaxed

For the next moment allow the muscles of your right shoulder to feel heavy and relaxed.

Next focus on your left shoulder, and silently in your mind repeat the following:

My left shoulder is heavy and relaxed
My left shoulder is heavy and relaxed

For the next moment allow the muscles of your left shoulder to feel heavy and relaxed.

[Perform the same sequence as you ask your clients to focus all their attention on the following]

- Left arm
- Right arm
- Left hand
- Right hand
- Left hip
- Right hip
- Left leg
- Right leg
- Left foot
- Right foot

Allow your mind to rest upon your chest, and silently in your mind repeat the following:

My breathing is easy and smooth
My breathing is easy and smooth

For the next few moments allow your breathing to be easy and smooth.

[If you wish you can repeat the above sequence, working through the body using the phrase 'warm and relaxed']

My left shoulder is warm and relaxed
My right shoulder is warm and relaxed etc.

Allow your whole body to feel warm, relaxed and easy. Repeat to yourself.

My whole body feels warm, relaxed and easy
My whole body feels warm, relaxed and easy

After a few seconds change this to:

*My whole body **is** warm, relaxed and easy*

Enjoy this feeling of relaxation you have created.

You feel very relaxed, softer and warm. Rest comfortably for a few minutes.

Become aware of the ground beneath you and the space around you. Come round slowly, gently stretching.

Slowly come into a sitting position.

SCRIPT FOR MEDITATION

Lie down on your back, or sit comfortably in the chair.

Take a few moments to get comfortable and let your body go heavy. Let the chair or floor or mat support the weight of your body completely.

Close your eyes, breathe easily and normally. Don't force your breathing. Concentrate on your breathing for a few moments.

Think of one word that you associate with being relaxed. The word may be something like 'calm', 'peaceful', 'sunshine' or even 'relaxed'.

Say the word silently to yourself each time you breathe out. Breathe in… breathe out… and say the word in your mind; breathe in… breathe out… and say the word in your mind.

Let yourself relax like this for about 10–15 minutes.

[When the relaxation time is completed bring the group back slowly and gently. Never jump up too quickly after a relaxation session.]

Become aware of the ground beneath you…
The space around you…
Come round slowly…
Gently stretching…
Slowly come into a sitting position.

INDEX